Health Informatics

This series is directed to healthcare professionals leading the transformation of healthcare by using information and knowledge. For over 20 years, Health Informatics has offered a broad range of titles: some address specific professions such as nursing, medicine, and health administration; others cover special areas of practice such as trauma and radiology; still other books in the series focus on interdisciplinary issues, such as the computer based patient record, electronic health records, and networked healthcare systems. Editors and authors, eminent experts in their fields, offer their accounts of innovations in health informatics. Increasingly, these accounts go beyond hardware and software to address the role of information in influencing the transformation of healthcare delivery systems around the world. The series also increasingly focuses on the users of the information and systems: the organizational, behavioral, and societal changes that accompany the diffusion of information technology in health services environments.

Developments in healthcare delivery are constant; in recent years, bioinformatics has emerged as a new field in health informatics to support emerging and ongoing developments in molecular biology. At the same time, further evolution of the field of health informatics is reflected in the introduction of concepts at the macro or health systems delivery level with major national initiatives related to electronic health records (EHR), data standards, and public health informatics.

These changes will continue to shape health services in the twenty-first century. By making full and creative use of the technology to tame data and to transform information, Health Informatics will foster the development and use of new knowledge in healthcare.

Brenda Kulhanek • Kathleen Mandato
Editors

Healthcare Technology Training

An Evidence-based Guide for Improved Quality

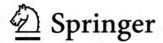
Springer

Editors
Brenda Kulhanek
School of Nursing
Vanderbilt University
Nashville, TN
USA

Kathleen Mandato
Vanderbilt University Medical Center
Nashville, TN
USA

ISSN 1431-1917   ISSN 2197-3741   (electronic)
Health Informatics
ISBN 978-3-031-10324-7   ISBN 978-3-031-10322-3   (eBook)
https://doi.org/10.1007/978-3-031-10322-3

This Springer imprint is published by the registered company Springer Nature Switzerland AG
The registered company address is: Gewerbestrasse 11, 6330 Cham, Switzerland

This book is dedicated to informatics nurses and other healthcare staff who tirelessly work to create engaging and effective training for health information technology—I have spent many years in your shoes! I also dedicate this book to my sweet husband Mark, who kept the home fires burning during the many months while I was busy writing.

Brenda Kulhanek

This book is dedicated in memory of my mom, Maureen Kelly Mandato, who served as a tremendous role model, friend, and faithful supporter. Thank you for teaching me to believe in myself and for always encouraging me to take risks and follow my dreams;

to Dirk Essary, thank you for all your endless support and encouragement;

to my amazing colleagues, Summer Warren, Stephanie Keene, Laura Meyer, Stacey Klein, and Mindy Parker. It is a true pleasure to work with you every day in the trenches to make a difference! Your commitment to always improving training motivates me to approach training in creative ways.

Kathleen Mandato

Foreword

Somewhere around mid-2006, I was faced with a dilemma. My young, recently established healthcare IT firm was providing education consulting resources to a large midwestern hospital system, and we began to be approached by other, non-education departments with consulting requests. We were at a crossroads. Would we branch out into all areas of healthcare IT, or would we stay true to our vision of becoming the go-to provider of learning services supporting mastery of technologies in clinical settings? The broader path seemed more lucrative but remaining specialized would allow us to hone our expertise in adult learning. I had particular interest in improving outcomes in EHR education—a rapidly expanding area that seemed to lack a clear, evidence-based methodology. Ultimately, I decided we would be most successful in achieving this by remaining exclusively a learning services firm within the healthcare market.

Did I make the right decision? I am now two decades into my career of providing education consulting resources and services to hospitals, and my honest answer may depend on the day you ask me. I feel blessed to be successful in a field that allows me to positively impact patient care—something I'm passionate about. But it hasn't been a path without frustration, as even today I find myself engaging healthcare executives in the same conversations I was having as "newbie" all those years ago. Within the wider healthcare arena, the need for quality healthcare IT education has historically been underestimated, and helping stakeholders understand why and how to prioritize education has not always been a linear process.

It could almost go without saying, then, that I am thrilled about *Healthcare Technology Training: An Evidence-based Guide for Improved Quality*, as my career has acquainted me with the great need for this text. This book takes readers through the theoretical underpinnings of adult learning through all faucets of its practical application to training in the healthcare environment. It covers what I hope that someday every informaticist understands about training. Instruction is supported by real-world examples from authors who have been tireless leaders in improving healthcare informatics education. Over the years, I have been fortunate to work personally with two of them: Linda Hainlen and Brenda Kulhanek.

I first met Linda in 2002 while she was Manager of Informatics Education at Clarian (now Indiana University) Health. At that time, I was a learning project manager working with the EHR vendor implementing at Clarian. It was Linda who first introduced me to the field of healthcare informatics. At the time, her education team was expected to simply take orders, responding to the cry of "we need this many people trained by this date." But Linda had a vision; she challenged her team to focus on the *desired outcomes* of the learning rather than the learning itself. She was the first person I heard suggest that we could improve clinical outcomes through better IT education, and she validated her assertion by introducing an iterative evaluation model that demonstrated whether outcomes were achieved. Over time, Linda was able to change the perception of her team from that of "order takers" to collaborative partners in achieving success.

My work with Clarian Health also led to my connection with Brenda Kulhanek. I first met Brenda when she was working as a nursing informatics specialist at Phoenix Children's Hospital. Later, she joined my consulting firm as a learning consultant for Clarian. There she embarked on a collaborative effort to support the improvement of provider education. It was in this role that Brenda first recognized the dearth of resources targeted at improving the quality of healthcare IT education. As her career has advanced through director and VP level positions within other healthcare organizations, she has maintained a deep commitment to elevating training programs through applying evidence-based learning approaches—a commitment that also led to her pursuit of advanced degrees in informatics, instructional design, and training. Now, after many years of experience, she has utilized her practical know-how and extensive theoretical grounding to create the healthcare training resource she has long wished was available.

Looking back at my start in providing healthcare learning services, it is hard to believe that firms dedicated to EHR and HIT education were nearly non-existent. It's even harder to believe healthcare informatics education is still neglected in many health systems and hospitals. Healthcare strives to be a 100% evidence-based industry, yet the quality of the healthcare IT training that we are asked to deliver is often limited by budget and time constraints. Given this difficult reality, how do we get back to—or even get started with—evidence-based informatics education? Answering this question is at the core of this text, and this is what makes it essential reading for anyone ready to begin a career in healthcare informatics, or anyone already in the field eager to transform their training to drive improved outcomes.

Sedona Learning Solutions   Kerry Kuehn
Phoenix, AZ, USA

Preface

Healthcare organizations are focused on providing evidence-based care to their patients, which includes health information technology. The delivery of patient care cannot be separated from technology, and informatics nurses are tasked with providing the training needed to effectively use new technology. Until now there has been a lack of resources available to help informatics nurses and other healthcare staff provide the evidence-based training that can improve the adoption and use of health information technology in the workplace, ultimately improving patient care.

This textbook has been written as a resource for informatics nurses so that they can use the same evidence that training professionals use to produce effective learning. We have gathered authors from multiple areas of practice to contribute to this book. Each informatics nurse and learning professional has gained unique training experiences, knowledge, and wisdom that provide a well-rounded approach to health information technology training. At the beginning of each chapter, we have included a short story or scenario to help illustrate the concepts presented in the following chapter text.

Nashville, TN   Brenda Kulhanek
Nashville, TN   Kathleen Mandato

Acknowledgments

After finding out that we graduated from the same university with a PhD (What a small world!), the start of a great partnership was formed, and I would like to acknowledge the wonderful teamwork with Dr. Mandato to write and co-edit this textbook.

We would also like to acknowledge the time and effort of our chapter authors. Your wisdom and experience have added a valuable and essential dimension to this textbook that will ultimately improve the delivery of healthcare.

About the Book

This book is divided into 15 chapters, each of which represent a part of the health information technology training process. To provide context, each chapter begins with a story or summary that illustrates the concept to be discussed in the chapter. Following each chapter, discussion questions provide a foundation for teaching and learning. Additionally, each chapter is supported with a presentation to guide instructors, and some chapters include templates and resources to add to the training toolkit for the learning audience.

Contents

About the Editors

Brenda Kulhanek is an associate professor at the Vanderbilt University School of Nursing. Her past professional roles include Division VP of Clinical Education for TriStar Health in Nashville, TN; corporate AVP of Clinical Education for HCA in Nashville, TN; corporate director of informatics at Adventist Health in Sacramento, CA; and nursing informatics specialist at Phoenix Children's Hospital in Phoenix, AZ. In addition, Dr. Kulhanek has served as an adjunct faculty for graduate-level nursing informatics for almost 10 years. Dr. Kulhanek holds a PhD from Capella University and is board certified in nursing informatics, nursing professional development, and nursing executive leadership. She was the president of the American Nursing Informatics Association from 2016 to 2017 and initiated several partnerships between ANIA and other organizations. Among her informatics publications and presentations are chapters in the Sigma Theta Tau nursing informatics textbook *Mastering Informatics: A Healthcare Handbook for Success*; the seventh edition of the *Handbook of Informatics for Nurses & Healthcare Professionals*; several modules of the Office of the National Coordinator (ONS) Workforce Development Program; two chapters in Nursing and Informatics for the twenty-first century; and as a workgroup member for the 2022 edition of the Nursing Informatics Scope and Standards publication. She teaches informatics at the master's and doctoral levels at Vanderbilt University and has a particular interest in strengthening nursing through nursing informatics education, and the integration of informatics into practice to support improvement of patient outcomes.

Kathleen Mandato is the Director of Epic Training & Delivery and the Administrative/Nursing Fellowship Program at Vanderbilt University Medical Center. She has worked in the field of training and organizational development since 1996; the telecommunications field from 1999 to 2005; and the healthcare industry since 2005. Kathleen has an MBA and a PhD in Education with a specialization in Training and Performance Improvement. She is a registered corporate coach and is Epic Software certified in the Cadence application. She serves as a member of the Trevecca Nazarene University Healthcare Advisory Council. Kathleen also teaches healthcare-related undergraduate/graduate classes as an adjunct professor. When not working, she enjoys movies, cooking, and traveling.

Chapter 1
The Importance of Training

Brenda Kulhanek and Kathleen Mandato

Abstract Understanding how to use training best practices can improve training outcomes and increase efficiency. It is important to meet the development needs of the health care workforce who take care of patients by providing effective and succinct training. The goal of this chapter is to introduce the importance of evidence-based practices for learning professionals. Evidence-based principles will be discussed throughout the book to help guide the management and delivery of high-quality training programs.

Keywords ADDIE · Evidence-based training · Best practices · Performance · Intervention

Learning Outcomes
1. Explain the importance of evidence-based training for organizational success
2. Discuss the difference between education and training
3. Describe the rationale for aligning training with the organizational mission and vision

B. Kulhanek
School of Nursing, Vanderbilt University, Nashville, TN, USA

K. Mandato (✉)
Epic Training & Delivery and Administrative/Nursing Fellowship Program, Vanderbilt University Medical Center, Nashville, TN, USA

B. Kulhanek, K. Mandato (eds.), *Healthcare Technology Training*, Health Informatics, https://doi.org/10.1007/978-3-031-10322-3_1

The Importance of Using Evidence-Based Training Methods

Shanice was tasked with creating the training for an upcoming health information technology implementation. She was part of the nursing informatics team and was very familiar with how the new technology would work, how it interfaced with other technology used in the hospital, and the decisions made when the technology was developed. However, Shanice did not have any guidance for how to create evidence-based training to prepare staff for the upcoming implementation. Based on past training experiences in the organization, and faced with a minimal training budget, Shanice created a 68-page presentation that went into great detail about every aspect of how the new technology would work once implemented. This document was printed and distributed to each nursing unit, where it sat on a table in the break room. Those nurses brave enough to look at the document quickly put it down after scanning just a few pages of information. As the implementation date drew closer, organizational leaders believed that all of the staff were getting the training they needed to effectively use the new health information technology system.

When the electronic health record (EHR) system was finally implemented, nursing leaders noted an immediate rise in late medication administrations, missed medications, medication errors, missed orders, treatments that were not delivered, and increased nursing dissatisfaction. Over the next few weeks overtime increased, hospital-acquired patient infections were on the rise, physicians expressed frustration with the EHR, nurses were taking more sick days, and some of the senior nurses turned in their resignations. Change can create turbulence within an organization, but how could an evidence-based approach to EHR training help to alleviate the negative impact of this change?

Introduction to Evidence-Based Training

Training is expensive. Care providers are removed from the work schedule and paid to attend class while a replacement care provider is paid to care for patients. Additionally, poor training can result in increased health care errors, decreased efficiency, patient dissatisfaction, and staff frustration. The purpose of this book is to provide a source of evidence-based best practices that informaticists and learning professionals can reference to develop and implement effective health information technology (HIT) training that best meets the needs of the learners who support patient care. Currently, there are minimal resources to guide evidence-based training for the informatics nurses and other health care staff tasked with developing and delivering HIT training. An understanding of training best practices, learning theories, and knowledge of the evidence that is used to guide training best practices can improve patient outcomes, decrease health care errors, and improve staff satisfaction. The goal of this book is to provide the knowledge needed to support a more confident and effective approach to delivering and managing training.

Learning professionals are able to produce consistent and high-quality training by consistently using evidence-based training methods. One of the most common training best practices is the ADDIE Model, which provides a robust framework for determining training needs, identifying interventions, and evaluating outcomes [1]. ADDIE stands for Analyze, Design, Develop, Implement and Evaluate, and each of the steps of the ADDIE model highlights the purpose of a training program. Every training program starts with a gap in knowledge or skills, referred to as a performance problem because without the proper knowledge and skills, staff cannot perform as expected with new technology. The ADDIE model assists training professionals to address performance problems by evaluating training from three different perspectives; the organizational perspective, team perspective, and individual employee perspective. The ADDIE Model will be covered in more detail in later chapters along with other frameworks used for structuring efficient and effective training content.

An additional important theme for learning professionals to consider is when and how to use training best practices, and knowing what to do and what to avoid when it comes to delivering effective training. Many times, this knowledge comes from experience gained through trial and error. Throughout this book, the authors will share their experience and wisdom by providing real-life examples that help illustrate the importance of evidence-based practice. Just as patient care delivery is based on evidence and best-practices, learning professionals can utilize established guidelines and evidence developed by other learning professionals to guide efficient and effective training programs.

To begin with, there are some general guiding principles that should be considered as essential when it comes to developing training. The first item is educating health care leaders, and reinforcing the importance of creating evidence-based training developed by using established frameworks and learning theories. Training must be structured in a way that best meets the needs of the learners. When a formal needs assessment is not conducted and established models are not used to fully understand performance issues, training will be less effective and may possibly focus on the wrong problem. An example of this is when learning professionals attempt to devise a *one size fits all* strategy to address a performance issue.

Although at first glance a one-size fits all training plan might appear to save money and resources, this strategy rarely works well and often causes learning professionals to lose credibility in the eyes of the learners and organization. Requiring learners to sit through a class to acquire information about a topic that they already know, or having them learn something that they will never use is a waste of time and resources. Following the correct steps of the ADDIE Model is essential to developing the right training for the right employee at the right time.

Training Is Not Always the Solution

It is important to use evidence and best practices when developing and delivering training, however, training is not always the correct solution to a performance problem. A thorough needs analysis can identify if the problem is technology related, workflow related, or associated with a behavioral issue. An example of a scenario when training was not the right solution is the following request. Leaders asked that a group of nurses undergo retraining on how to use an EHR communication process correctly. The identified problem was that messages created by the nurses were not being saved to the patient's chart. In this case, leaders decided that the nurses were doing something wrong and the initial solution was to require the nurses to go back through training. Training is often the first solution proposed by leaders when a critical problem arises. After analysis, the real issue in this case was identified as a system problem that randomly caused some messages to not be saved. Without a needs assessment, unnecessary time and resources would have been devoted to an issue that had nothing to do with training. In addition, unnecessary training can be viewed as a punitive action with a decrease in staff morale [2].

There are times when an informal training solution may be the best method to meet the needs of the learners. After performing a needs assessment, and following the steps of the ADDIE Model, it may be determined that creating a job aide, or tip sheet is the best solution for demonstrating a recent change in the EHR system. An informal style of training may be the best solution for smaller changes, especially if the learners are already familiar with the system. Understanding the audience and selecting the correct type of training is essential to providing effective training.

The previous examples have illustrated the importance of following evidence-based practices when it comes to providing training solutions. Awareness of the performance issue and knowledge of the learning audience is key to establishing a robust training program. When first implementing evidence-based training, it may take some time for the entire team of learning professionals to incorporate these evidence-based training practices so that they become part of a standard procedure for the entire training group. Once training best practices are in place, the next challenge will be to establish a routine for partnering with health care leaders and stakeholders to implement evidence-based change.

Reinforcing the role of the training team as a formal partner in providing organizational solutions will help solidify the partnership and build commitment among leaders. In subsequent chapters, information about creating a culture where training is a regular part of ongoing efforts to implement successful changes within the organization will be presented. As evidence-based training practices are incorporated into an organization and training outcomes improve, the use of evidence-based training practices will build credibility for the training team.

Education Versus Training

Many people use the terms *education* and *training* interchangeably. How these terms are defined and understood impacts the entire process of designing, developing, and delivering training. The purpose of training is to develop skills in order to perform a task. The goal of education is to obtain knowledge [3]. To further highlight the difference between education and training, would a bakery be more

Fig. 1.1 Education vs. training

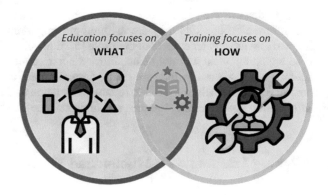

successful if the baker has undergone education about pastries, or has obtained hands-on training to make pastries? In reality, education and training can be intertwined, or the process of training can lead to education when more knowledge is desired (see Fig. 1.1). Conversely, education can include training so that both knowledge and skills are developed, this is often seen in simulation labs for nurses and nursing students [4].

Understanding the difference between training and education is important because it drives the approach used to design and deliver new skills or knowledge. When an educational approach is employed, the focus of the activity will be on providing information and knowledge to learners. The educational outcome is for the learner to leave the course with new knowledge. In nursing, examples of education could include a class on the function of the liver, new care approaches for diabetic patients, or information about how to assess for suicide risk in a patient. These courses do not include a hands-on component and a large portion of didactic courses in colleges and universities are examples of education rather than training.

On the other hand, the focus of training is to exit the course with the ability to perform a new skill or task. The training approach includes opportunities for hands-on practice so that learners can perform in a real-world environment after training is completed. Examples of training classes for nurses include simulation with manikins, performing a new wound care technique on a simulator, learning to tie patient restraints in a lab, or developing the skill to use health information technology (HIT). However, HIT training without interspersed education that presents the purpose for each process will result in a skills-only approach that will not fully meet the needs of the learning audience, or attain the quality outcomes needed in healthcare.

Because training is primarily skills focused, the training audience may be grouped by those who will use the same skills and processes in their daily work. This means that unit secretaries might attend one HIT class focused on the activities found in their daily work, nursing leaders may attend a class focused on different information and processes that align with their roles, and patient care nurses on a specific unit may receive training that includes only what is essential to know to perform their daily work.

Regardless of the educational approach, adult learners value understanding why the information or skills they are learning are important, and to interpret what is learned into the greater context of their role [5]. Education or knowledge that is delivered without context will not be useful for a nurse or other healthcare provider, and training that does not include the context, the purpose, and the importance of each step in a process will not provide reliable adherence to the new processes. Further information about learning theories and brain science will be presented in Chap. 5.

Aligning Training with Mission and Vision

In the nursing profession, the most current evidence and best practices are used to guide the care provided to patients. This information is available to nurses and healthcare workers through written policies, guidelines embedded in the electronic health record, and scholarly databases that can be accessed with the click of the mouse. In light of all of the focus on using evidence-based resources available to nurses and other caregivers for the best provision of healthcare, are we using the most current best practices and evidence to guide the development and delivery of health information technology training?

In subsequent chapters, evidence and best-practices from the training industry will be presented to provide the foundations for HIT training programs that support each organizational mission and vision by producing training that is not only more efficient, but also more effective at generating learning outcomes that can help healthcare providers to utilize technology in a more effective manner. When health care providers are adequately trained to use HIT, patient privacy is supported, and patient care is safer and of a higher quality [6, 7]. HIT has been widely used in healthcare for nearly a decade, yet studies continue to highlight the impact of poor training on patient outcomes, nursing satisfaction, healthcare quality and safety, patient satisfaction, and the validity of reportable healthcare data [8–12].

When a training program is developed, it is important to align the program with the organizational mission and vision. Aligning training with the mission ensures that leaders in the organization are supportive of the training program. In addition, if training is aligned with the mission, the organizational mission can be embedded into the training content so that learners can clearly see how the changes being presented in training align with the mission and help support or grow this mission. This alignment with strategy is important so that learners can clearly see that a change, which may feel threatening to the staff, is intended to help the organization continue to more forward according to their mission.

Aligning training with the mission and vision also requires alignment and involvement of organizational leaders. It is no secret that the implementation of health information technology can often trigger resistance and frustration among healthcare staff. Involvement of leaders can help to provide endorsement of the training at the highest levels, and positive messages in support of the training often provide benefits that can help guide acceptance of the change.

Why Is Training Important?

As changes take place in the work environment and technology advances, there will always be a need for employees to understand and align with these changes through development of their knowledge and skills. Training professionals and their teams provide a valuable service in helping employees develop their skill sets so they can adapt to changes and be more efficient in performing their jobs. When employees feel confident about doing their job because they possess the proper knowledge and skills, they become more productive and add greater value to the organization. Another benefit of training is that employees who are confident deliver better results and improved outcomes for the organization.

Nurses and other clinical staff benefit from training every day as they take care of their patients. They rely on training to show them the correct process for taking care of patients and documenting in the EHR. Training is essential in helping to prevent errors and reduce adverse incidents that affect patient care. Without the proper training, clinical staff can put their patients at risk as well as put themselves at risk. When nurses and other clinical staff possess the proper training and know where to find training resources as they need them, they become better equipped to handle change and take care of their patients. Increased skills as delivered through effective training give staff the knowledge and ability to do their jobs, reducing stress, burnout, and increasing employee satisfaction. Additionally, when a patient receives confident care from a well-trained healthcare provider, patients feel that they are receiving good care which often helps with recovery.

Summary

Today's health information technology is complex, and EHR training is essential for providing safe patient care. Nurses and other clinical staff use the EHR and other technology every day to document care, and technology cannot be separated from clinical care. It is critical that staff receive the most effective training on how to use health information technology based on their role. The EHR contains the information needed to provide safe patient care. Information within the EHR is considered the facility's legal record of the treatment course provided to patients, and the patient's response to treatment. It therefore becomes critical that the data entered in the EHR record is accurate and complete. Learning professionals play an important part in training and preparing clinical staff to use the medical record and other health information technology safely and effectively. Insufficient training can lead to missing information, medical errors, and produce unreliable data that can place the organization and patient in jeopardy.

Training is a key element in employee satisfaction and engagement. When employees feel that the organization that they are working for is investing in them, they become more motivated and engaged. Training helps with instilling confidence and building proficiency. It also promotes continuous improvement and learning opportunities that can provide career development and growth over time. All these elements help to enhance the employee experience and create loyalty and retention.

Discussion Questions and Answers

1. Learning professionals are able to produce consistent and high-quality training by using evidence-based training methods. Which model/method was discussed in Chap. 1? Why it is important?

   One of the most common training best practices is the ADDIE Model, which provides a robust framework for determining training needs, identifying interventions, and evaluating outcomes. The ADDIE model assists training professionals to address performance problems by evaluating training from three different perspectives; the organizational perspective, team perspective, and individual employee perspective.

2. Why is it important to use evidence-based practices when developing training?

   It is important to use evidence-based practices because they provide a framework to use for conducting a needs analysis to determine the root cause of a problem. In some cases, training may be the recommended solution and in other cases a non-training intervention may be required.

3. What is the difference between training and education?

   When an educational approach is employed, the focus of the activity will be on providing information and knowledge to learners. The educational outcome is for the learner to leave the course with new knowledge. On the other hand, the focus of training is to exit the course with the ability to perform a new skill or task. The training approach includes opportunities for hands-on practice so that learners can perform in a real-world environment after training is completed.

4. Why is it important to align a training program with the organizational mission and vision?

   Aligning training with the mission ensures that leaders in the organization are supportive of the training program. In addition, if training is aligned with the mission, the organizational mission can be embedded into the training content so that learners can clearly see how the changes being presented in training align with the mission and support or grow this mission.

References

1. Nair SR (2017) *Using the Addie model to create effective training interventions.* Retrieved October 10, 2021 from https://www.linkedin.com/pulse/using-addie-model-create-effective-training-sajan-nair
2. Wright D. The ultimate guide to competency assessment in health care. Creative Health Care Management; 2005.
3. Katsikas S. Health care management and information systems security: awareness, training or education? Int J Med Inform. 2000;60(2):129–35. https://doi.org/10.1016/s1386-5056(00)00112-x.

4. Vecchione A. Practical education: a nursing simulation lab offers efficient, cost-effective train-ing. NJBIZ. 2019;32(6):9–11.
5. Knowles MS, Holton EF III, Swanson RA. The adult learner: the definitive classic in adult education and human resources development. 6th ed. Elsevier Butterworth Heinemann; 2005.
6. Kisekka V, Giboney JS. The effectiveness of health care information technologies: evaluation of trust, security beliefs, and privacy as determinants of health care outcomes. J Med Internet Res. 2018;20(4):e107. https://doi.org/10.2196/jmir.9014.
7. Strawn JA. Maintaining registered nurses' currency in informatics. Las Vegas: University of Nevada; 2017.
8. Colicchio TK, Cimino JJ, Fiol GD, Del Fiol G. Unintended consequences of Nationwide elec-tronic health record adoption: challenges and opportunities in the post-meaningful use era. J Med Internet Res. 2019;21:6), N.PAG-N.PAG. https://doi.org/10.2196/13313.
9. McBride S, Tietze M, Robichaux C, Stokes L, Weber E. Identifying and addressing ethical issues with use of electronic health records. Online J Issues Nurs. 2018;23(1):6–6. https://doi.org/10.3912/OJIN.Vol23No01Man05.
10. Meyerhoefer CD, Sherer SA, Deily ME, Chou S-Y, Guo X, Chen J, Sheinberg M, Levick D. Provider and patient satisfaction with the integration of ambulatory and hospital EHR sys-tems. J Am Med Inform Assoc. 2018;25(8):1054–63. https://doi.org/10.1093/jamia/ocy048.
11. Olivares Bøgeskov B, Grimshaw-Aagaard SLS. Essential task or meaningless burden? Nurses' perceptions of the value of documentation. Nordic J Nurs Res. 2019;39(1):9–19. https://doi.org/10.1177/2057158518773906.
12. Schoenbaum A, & Carroll W (2020) *Nursing informatics key role in defining clini-cal workflow, increasing efficiency and improving quality.* HIMSS Resource Center: Informatics. Retrieved October 10, 2021 from https://www.himss.org/resources/nursing-informatics-key-role-defining-clinical-workflow-increasing-efficiency-and

Brenda Kulhanek is an associate professor at the Vanderbilt University School of Nursing and has a history of leadership in both informatics and clinical education. Dr. Kulhanek holds a PhD from Capella University and a doctor of nursing practice (DNP) from Walden University. She is board certified in nursing informatics, nursing professional development, and executive leadership. Her publications include informatics textbook chapters and multiple informatics articles. She recently participated in the Scope & Standards for Nursing Informatics publication. She teaches informatics at the master's and doctoral levels and has a particular interest in strengthening nursing through nursing informatics education, and the integration of informatics into practice to support improvement of patient outcomes.

Kathleen Mandato is the Director of Epic Training & Delivery and the Administrative/Nursing Fellowship Program at Vanderbilt University Medical Center. She has worked in the field of train-ing and organizational development for the last twenty-seven years; ten years in telecommunica-tions, and seventeen years in the healthcare industry. Kathleen has an MBA and a PhD in Education with a specialization in Training & Performance Improvement. She is a registered corporate coach and is Epic Software certified in the Cadence application. Kathleen also teaches healthcare related undergraduate/graduate classes as an Adjunct Professor at Trevecca Nazarene and Cumberland Universities.

Chapter 2
The Impact of Inadequate Training

Kathleen Mandato and Brenda Kulhanek

Abstract Effective training provides a solid foundation for accessing patient information and documentation of patient care. Medical errors can be directly attributed to a lack of training to use technology. In addition, a lack of confidence and extra work effort are often the results of inadequate or rushed health information technology training. To create a successful training program, training professionals must take into consideration different learning needs as well as acknowledge previous knowledge and experience. By investing time upfront, training professionals can develop the right formula that works for the training team and the organization.

Keywords Health information technology (HIT) · Electronic health record (EHR) Effective training · Technology · Efficiency · Inadequate training

Learning Outcomes
1. Discuss the relationship between inadequate training and patient care
2. List three potential consequences of inadequate training
3. Evaluate the ethical foundation for adequate training
4. Plan methods to justify evidence-based training

K. Mandato (✉)
Epic Training & Delivery and Administrative/Nursing Fellowship Program, Vanderbilt University Medical Center, Nashville, TN, USA

B. Kulhanek
School of Nursing, Vanderbilt University, Nashville, TN, USA

B. Kulhanek, K. Mandato (eds.), *Healthcare Technology Training*, Health Informatics, https://doi.org/10.1007/978-3-031-10322-3_2

The Many Consequences of Inadequate Training

Jack worked in a hospital where a new EHR system was being implemented to replace the current system. Because the patient care staff were familiar with using an EHR system, organizational leaders decided to provide abbreviated training to save on training costs. Short video clips were created to show processes in the workflow of the new EHR, and each video clip contained a single process such as how to view and acknowledge orders in one video, or how to document medications in another video. The learners were emailed a lengthy document that outlined the technical aspects of every function in the system, however, the document was written as a technical manual and few staff took the time to read through 154 pages of information. When the new system was implemented, leaders noted that hospital-acquired infection rates were rising, medication errors increased, the number of mislabeled lab specimens increased, and nurses were increasingly frustrated.

What happened to cause this sudden shift in organizational outcomes and nursing attitudes? Due to inadequate training with the new EHR system, the nurses were not able to confidently locate information such as when an IV or central line dressing was last changed, or the length of time a urinary catheter had been in place. In addition, a bar code scanning system for medication administration and lab specimens was implemented during the change to the new EHR system. Because nurses felt that the bar code scanning process was too cumbersome, they started using workarounds that did not include the bar code scanner. Many nurses were leaving work at the end of the shift feeling exhausted from caring for their patients while struggling to find and enter information into a new EHR.

The Impact of Inadequate Training

Medical errors still occur, even when using health information technology (HIT). The nature of these errors is often directly related to a lack of training to use the technology [1, 2]. The cost of medical errors may impact a health care organization far more than the cost of providing high quality, effective training. In addition to errors of omission and commission made while using HIT, data obtained from an EHR system may not be valid and reliable if not entered into the correct locations in the system, or may not be entered at all.

Although medical errors were present long before the EHR was incorporated into healthcare, effective HIT training provides a solid foundation for documentation of patient care that can deter a lawsuit [3]. As more documentation is moving into an electronic format, the frequency of lawsuits has decreased [4], yet a lack of training has been a factor as the root cause of many errors and near misses [5].

Another impact of inadequate training can create a lack of confidence that results in the care provider focused more on the computer than on the patient [6]. When care providers are adequately trained to use the EHR, they demonstrate more confidence in using the technology which results in increased and higher quality patient interactions. When patients and their families have high quality interactions and communication with caregivers, the amount of patient learning, compliance with treatment, and ratings of their care increase [7]. Finally, when nurses and other caregivers are not adequately trained to use HIT, the quality of data retrieved from the EHR system declines. As an example, a hospital was implementing a new nursing documentation system. The nurses and other caregivers underwent training that included basic system functionality but did not include adequate explanations about why certain processes and workflows functioned the way that they did. Within 48 h of implementation, a few of the nurses found a workaround for patient care documentation so that they could avoid using the multiple pick-lists in the system to document their assessments. Within another 36 h, almost every caregiver was documenting using this workaround. The consequence of this workaround was that no patient assessment data was flowing into other areas of the chart to guide treatment plans, orders, or to evaluate outcomes. In this case, and in many other cases where training does not address the use of workarounds or prevent documenting in incorrect locations in the EHR, patient care is negatively impacted. Data obtained from the EHR during that period of 4 days was inaccurate and could have led to errors in treatments and orders.

The Ethical Responsibilities of Training

According to the ANA Code of Ethics [8], nurses are responsible to promote patient safety, reduce errors, and maintain a culture of safety. They are responsible first to the patient, as the recipient of health care services. This code of ethics holds true both for informatics nurses and others who develop EHR training to ensure that the training outcomes will result in the highest levels of safety and quality for patient care. The code of ethics additionally applies to the learners receiving EHR training. Learning professionals, even with the most engaging training design, may need to remind the caregiver participants that they have an ethical responsibility to their patients to learn the EHR system so that they can utilize the tools of technology to provide quality patient care.

The Impact of Inadequate Training on Staff

Training has a significant impact on the organization and the ability for clinical staff to effectively use an EHR. When employees do not receive adequate training, they often make up for it by fumbling through the system doing what they perceive to be correct, which is probably not correct. The other option for system users who are confused is to ask a co-worker who probably does not know either, and may leave out important information. All of this leads to tremendous stress and frustration on the part of the user, which in turn impacts patient satisfaction and care. It is critical that employees receive adequate training by learning professionals who can guide them in how to use the medical record effectively based on their role and scope. In many cases, there is a tremendous push to expedite the onboarding and training processes for nurses and other staff so that they can help alleviate staffing needs on the patient care units. Shortchanging these employees and preventing them from attending a full training event with built in practice time provides them a great disservice. The lack of confidence and extra work effort that results from insufficient training leads to decreased morale, potential loss of revenue, not to mention the potential impact for adverse patient care.

System rejection is another ramification of improper, or inadequate training. When clinical staff do not know how to use the system properly, they often do not use the system very efficiently. Over time, this leads to a great deal of frustration and rejection of the system itself [9]. It takes time to acclimate to a medical record system and effective training can help patient care staff to more quickly acclimate to technology.

Because HIT systems are complex, an option is to provide basic training to clinical staff so that they can safely use the system. At a later date the staff can experience additional optimization training where they learn to use the system more efficiently with enhanced capabilities. For organizations to adequately prepare their staff, they must invest in the proper training programs to prepare their staff for success. There also must be a policy in place that guides the requirements of training because training should not be an afterthought or optional. Training should be integrated as a core piece of the mission of the organization. Without proper training, patients and staff will suffer and the organization may experience a negative financial impact. Leadership must endorse policies that requires training before staff can receive access to the EHR. For example, doctors and nurses are not allowed to practice medicine without completing the proper training and passing the necessary exams. Likewise, all staff should be required to complete the proper role-based training before being allowed to access and document in the medical record, which is a repository of all documentation and interpretation of care provided to the patient. *No training, no access no kidding* should be the mantra adopted in each organization. Considering staffing and budgetary pressures, it is important to have the commitment of leaders in helping to reinforce this policy.

Drivers of Training Need

Technology is at the heart of all that we do to help take care of patients, and at this time technology cannot be separated from clinical care. We use technology every day to help people, and in the process further develop our knowledge base and implement innovative processes to attain greater efficiency. Therefore, it is not surprising that technology is often used to deliver training. Technology can provide the means to show how to effectively use the medical record. Online training modules or training environments can be used to illustrate what a patient's record would look like in the real world.

Technology is a wonderful tool, but it does not guarantee the success of training or positive patient outcomes. Technology should support patient care and allow the focus to be on the patient. The goal should not be about the technology but rather using that technology to provide better care for the patient. It is important for health information technologies to be designed with patient-oriented workflows in mind instead of just focusing on the tasks to be completed. Likewise, training should focus on the overall processes and functionality of the medical record that will lead to effective management of healthcare information for the patient.

Training is an essential ingredient to the success of any organization. Employees who are trained well gain new knowledge and skills that they can use to increase efficiency and potentially reduce costs in the workplace. Investing in training upfront saves a lot of time and money down the road. Employees need to be oriented and trained up front to understand what is expected of them as well as to help them be successful in their new role. To create a successful training program, learning professionals must take into consideration different learning needs as well as acknowledge the previous knowledge and experience of the learning audience. Offering a test down option can help evaluate the knowledge levels of new employees with previous experience; and can potentially save time and money by not training employees on what they already know.

Learners differ in how they take in information and process it. As training professionals, it is important to offer multiple methods of learning based on different tools and techniques that help engage the learner. With multiple variables to consider, a one-size-fits-all solution rarely works. By investing time upfront, training professionals can develop the right formula that works for the training team and the organization. We will cover in subsequent chapters more details on the various tools and techniques that can help create effective training programs.

Many times, leaders in health care organizations push to shorten the length of HIT training in order to maximize nursing resources and cut training costs. However, when the costs and potential risks of inadequate EHR training are weighed against the expense of adequate and well-designed thorough EHR training, the additional cost of providing well-designed EHR training far outweighs the costs of patient care errors, nursing overtime, decreased patient satisfaction, and nursing burnout.

Discussion Questions and Answers

1. Why is Health Information Technology (HIT) training so important for patient care?

    Effective HIT training provides a solid foundation for documentation of patient care that can deter a lawsuit. A lack of training has an impact as the root cause of many errors and near misses. HIT can help provide more confidence in providers using technology to take care of patients. When nurses and other caregivers are not adequately trained to use HIT, the quality of data retrieved from the EHR system declines.

2. What is required to create a successful training program?

    To create a successful training program, training professionals must take into consideration different learning styles as well as acknowledge previous knowledge and experience. Offering a test down option can help evaluate the knowledge levels of new employees with previous experience; and can potentially save time and money by not training employees on what they already know. Learners differ in how they take in information and process it. As training professionals, it is important to offer multiple methods of learning based on different tools and techniques that help engage the learner.

3. What are some of the unanticipated consequences of inadequate HIT training?

Answer: The anticipated consequences of inadequate HIT training are a lack of confidence and extra work effort. In addition, there is low morale, potential loss of revenue, and the potential impact for adverse patient care. When clinical staff do not know how to use the system properly, they often do not use the system very efficiently. Over time, this leads to a great deal of frustration and rejection of the system.

References

1. Devin J, Cleary BJ, Cullinan S. The impact of health information technology on prescribing errors in hospitals: a systematic review and behaviour change technique analysis. Syst Rev. 2020;9:1. https://doi.org/10.1186/s13643-020-01510-7.
2. Furukawa MF. Electronic health record adoption and rates of in-hospital adverse events. J Patient Saf. 2020;16(2):137.
3. Hicks TC, Beck DE. Medical legal issues. In: Improving outcomes in colon and rectal surgery. CRC Press; 2018. p. 141–7.
4. Sharma L, Queenan C, Ozturk O. The impact of information technology and communication on medical malpractice lawsuits. Prod Oper Manag. 2019;28(10):2552–72.
5. Claffey C. Near-miss medication errors provide a wake-up call. Nursing2020. 2018;48(1):53–5.
6. Alkureishi MA, Lee WW, Lyons M, Wroblewski K, Farnan JM, Arora VM. Electronic-clinical evaluation exercise (e-CEX): a new patient-centered EHR use tool. Patient Educ Couns. 2018;101(3):481–9.
7. Arungwa OT. Effect of communication on nurse—patient relationship in national orthopaedic hospital, Igbobi, Lagos. West African J Nurs. 2014;25(2):37–49.
8. ANA (2015). *Code of ethics for nurses with interpretive statements.* nursesbooks.org.
9. Vitari C, Ologeanu-Taddei R. The intention to use an electronic health record and its antecedents among three different categories of clinical staff. BMC Health Serv Res. 2018;18:1–1. https://doi.org/10.1186/s12913-018-3022-0.

Kathleen Mandato is the Director of Epic Training & Delivery and the Administrative/Nursing Fellowship Program at Vanderbilt University Medical Center. She has worked in the field of training and organizational development for the last twenty-seven years; ten years in telecommunications, and seventeen years in the healthcare industry. Kathleen has an MBA and a PhD in Education with a specialization in Training & Performance Improvement. She is a registered corporate coach and is Epic Software certified in the Cadence application. Kathleen also teaches healthcare related undergraduate/graduate classes as an Adjunct Professor at Trevecca Nazarene and Cumberland Universities.

Brenda Kulhanek is an associate professor at the Vanderbilt University School of Nursing and has a history of leadership in both informatics and clinical education. Dr. Kulhanek holds a PhD from Capella University and a doctor of nursing practice (DNP) from Walden University. She is board certified in nursing informatics, nursing professional development, and executive leadership. Her publications include informatics textbook chapters and multiple informatics articles. She recently participated in the Scope & Standards for Nursing Informatics publication. She teaches informatics at the master's and doctoral levels and has a particular interest in strengthening nursing through nursing informatics education, and the integration of informatics into practice to support improvement of patient outcomes.

Chapter 3
Engaging Leaders

Renee Robinson

Abstract Leaders within a healthcare organization have a large impact on effective training delivery and the successful implementation of health information technology. Leaders create a culture that supports the success of a project, or leaders can create a culture that creates barriers for a project. Leaders are key stakeholders in moving a learning project from an initial vision to the final achievement of a goal. There are many different leadership styles, and this chapter addresses the role of the leader and the importance of becoming familiar with how to work with each type of leader to help facilitate the work of the learning professional and achieve project success.

Keywords Transactional · Transformational · Democratic · Autocratic' laisse-faire

Learning Outcomes
1. Describe the importance of leadership engagement in HIT training projects
2. Explain the impact of leadership style on project communication
3. Discuss the role of the informatics nurse as a leader when managing HIT training

---

R. Robinson (✉)
Ambulatory Clinical Informatics, LifeBridge Health, Baltimore, MD, USA

© The Author(s), under exclusive license to Springer Nature
Switzerland AG 2022
B. Kulhanek, K. Mandato (eds.), *Healthcare Technology Training*, Health
Informatics, https://doi.org/10.1007/978-3-031-10322-3_3

The Importance of Leadership Support

A large healthcare organization on the east coast was moving from paper to electronic charting. As part of the preparation process, the staff from each of the three regional hospitals were required to attend an off-site kick-off meeting. The purpose of the kickoff meeting was to share the details of the upcoming change to the staff. The meetings were scheduled so that staff could attend at a time that fit into their schedules. During each of these meetings, the health system executive, who was also the project sponsor, presented an eloquent message that stressed the importance of reducing patient harm by moving from paper to an electronic health record. The message of this leader was so empowering and heartfelt that staff left each meeting feeling inspired and empowered to make this difficult change. In this example, the leader was able to impact the natural anxiety that emerges around an unknown change, and build a strong, positive change culture focused on patient safety.

Introduction: The Importance of Leadership Engagement

The leaders within an organization have a great impact on both the delivery of health information technology (HIT) training and the success of the technology implementation. Leaders not only provide the resources for effective training, but also create a culture that supports the success of a project. An effective leader or leadership team empowers their staff to move from a vision to the successful achievement of a goal. However, there are many different styles of leadership and becoming familiar with how to work with each type of leader will help to facilitate the work of training and ultimately the final success of a project. This chapter will focus on the importance of leadership engagement, the impact a technology implementation can have on an organization, and the role of the training team and informatics nurse in implementing HIT training.

Leadership engagement with any HIT projects is imperative, and their engagement must extend beyond the scope of implementation to creating a supportive culture for training. The implementation of HIT represents a very large expenditure and implementation of very costly technology projects have failed due to poor training [1]. However, not all leaders recognize the importance of a solid training approach and one of the roles of the training team is to ensure that leaders are not only engaged, but also educated and aware of the importance of training.

Each major implementation project will have an executive sponsor, and the chief nursing executive is often the executive sponsor for HIT implementations that impact nursing. When working on an HIT training project, the first task for the learning professional is to engage with the leaders by identifying and connecting with the project sponsor as early as possible in the training plan process. It will be important to ensure that the project sponsor is fully aware of the identified training needs and the proposed training plan. The sponsor will be able to help remove barriers to effective training, and may engage additional leaders to facilitate the success of the training effort. When a project sponsor is not fully aware of the scope and needs of a project they will not be able to provide the resources and remove barriers that impact training success. When leaders and sponsors are not informed and engaged, it can have a detrimental impact on the training project [2].

Leadership Styles

When working with a project sponsor or leader, it is important to approach the leader in a way that best matches their leadership style and leadership language. For example, an autocratic leader will want to know more details about an HIT implementation than a transformational leader may want to know. Leadership styles can have an impact on project success, and almost all leadership styles can be seen within a single organization. There are no perfect leadership styles, and no leadership style represents good or bad leadership. However, understanding the basics of each leadership style will provide insight into how to approach the leader in an ongoing relationship.

Transactional Leaders

Transactional leaders persuade their followers by exchanging rewards for the services rendered, or consequences for failures. The transactional leader focuses on providing something in return when a task or action is accomplished for them.

Transformational Leaders

Transformational leaders use persuasion to get others to buy into their vision. This type of leader is charismatic in delivering their vision, resulting in staff empowerment. Empowerment increases staff engagement towards their work. Being productive at work is a choice and being empowered makes that choice even easier. When the leader is aware of and supports a vision, the transformational leadership style is often beneficial for HIT implementations.

Democratic Leadership

Democratic leadership is a shared decision-making model in which everyone participates in the decision-making process. The leaders may often provide the final approval on decisions, but every member of the team is involved in the decision-making process. The democratic leadership style is great for solving complex problems and connecting people to their work. However, the democratic leadership process can often delay decision-making due to the extensive involvement of all stakeholders.

Laissez-Faire Leadership

Laissez-faire leadership is a hands-off type of leadership that reactively engages the leader most often during times of crisis. This type of leadership style does not engage in micromanaging staff, trusting employees to be creative to get the work done without any direction, as long as it doesn't interfere with organizational operations. A hands-off leadership style may bring risk to an HIT project if key details or processes are omitted through lack of involvement.

Autocratic Leadership

Autocratic leadership is an authoritarian style where one person makes all the decisions without receiving any input. This leadership style lacks open and honest communication and when a leader uses an autocratic style, it is important that they are very knowledgeable about the HIT project details.

When communicating with a leader or project sponsor, the most successful transactions occur when the learning professional is aware of the communication style of the leader, based on their leadership style. If the style of communication does not align with a sponsor or leader's communication style, they may tune out the communication or only receive parts of the message. Table 3.1 outlines the different leadership styles and the best communication approaches for each type of leadership style.

The engagement of leaders is essential for successful HIT training, and without effective communication and support, an HIT implementation may not reach the full potential anticipated from the technology, or may have a greater chance of failure. However, not all leaders in health care are familiar with health information technology nor understand the importance of high-quality training to the success of an HIT implementation. Additionally, leaders are under pressure to maintain a project budget that is within scope, and are often the first ones to receive complaints about the HIT implementation. It is important to not only provide the information about how training will be planned and implemented, but also to share the importance of training and the relationship between training and successful outcomes.

Table 3.1 Relating to different leadership styles

Leadership Style	Description	Best communication approach
Transactional	Exchange of rewards for services rendered	Prefer limited communication, feedback may be delayed. Uses rewards to maintain engagement [3]. Uses consequences to discourage failure [4].
Transformational	Persuades others to buy into the vision and empowers staff to improve performance	Demonstrate autonomy [3]. Focus on alignment of activities with vision, mission, and goals. Transactional leaders identify with internalization of the vision [5]. Seek to build confidence and personal accountability [4].
Democratic	All members of the team share in decision-making	Welcomes team participation in decision-making [4]. Leaders are interested in discussion and consensus, prefer for planning to be completed by the team, but open to discussion and shared decision-making [6]
Laissez-faire	Hands-off leadership style that empowers employees to become creative to get work done	Prefers team to assume responsibility for decision-making [4]. Response to communication is typically passive unless serious problems arise. It may take extra effort to engage the leader in solving problems before they become serious [7]
Autocratic	The leader makes all decisions without input from the staff	Prefers to have complete control over decision making [4]. Wants to be involved in developing the rules and processes and to be in charge of enforcing how the work is done, exhibits limited flexibility in changing their opinions on how things should be done [6]

The Importance of Stakeholders

Stakeholders are those who will be impacted by the HIT project and can include physicians, nurses, laboratory staff, ancillary, managers, and more. Trainers are also stakeholders because the trainer's work is impacted by a project implementation. When presented with barriers or challenges, health organizations have executives or leaders available to assist with moving obstacles the can impeded the success of the HIT implementation.

During the early phases of a project, stakeholders will be impacted by decisions that are made about implementation of training, including when, where, and how training will take place. Additionally, when the training schedule is developed it will span across all clinicians, including ancillary staff. It will be critical to include leaders from all stakeholder groups when planning for the training program and implementation. Organizational and clinical leaders will want to achieve a workable schedule that will have little to no interruptions in day-to-day operations, including the time to fill open spots in schedules well before training occurs. If open staffing spots are not addressed, staff may be required to skip training to perform patient care, especially when events such as a pandemic produce a staff shortage or high patient volumes.

Depending on the staff population being trained for the new HIT system, there may be individuals with limited basic computer skills. If lack of basic computer skills is not addressed prior to training, staff will struggle to keep up with the rest of the class. In fact, lack of basic computer skills in the learner audience can interrupt or derail a training class. Consider offering classes in basic computer skills prior to a major HIT implementation so that staff without computer experience have a chance to learn computer functions and gain some time to practice. Adding additional training classes to address lagging technical skills can impact the budget and it will be important to keep leaders aware of project changes such as this. Additionally, anticipated class length may need to be adjusted if there are staff that lack typing skills, these learners may need a bit of extra time to complete learning activities that require keyboard skills.

HIT Training and the Impact on Operations

Training for the implementation of a HIT project is one the most important activities that facilitates project success. The biggest impact that HIT training has on the operations of an organization is financial. Each organization must train staff while keeping operations running, which requires extra staffing and an increased labor budget. Organizational leaders and sponsors will need to be involved in training plans in order to make the decisions necessary to train staff with minimal to no interruptions to operations.

One of the biggest decisions made by leaders is whether or not to make attending training mandatory for staff. Mandated training has direct positive impact on the success of a project, but this requires an organization to ask overstretched employees to find time in their busy day to attend training. The result of this is sometimes obvious, employees will put off learning the new HIT system for as long as they can in favor of keeping the status quo. In addition to mandating training, leaders will need to identify repercussions and consequences for not attending the mandatory training classes. The downside of not mandating training is that staff will perceive the training as less important, and will avoid attending classes. At that point, leaders have no ability to force staff to attend training.

Training can make or break the success of a go-live and even when mandated, staff will try to avoid attending class until the very last minute. Sometimes learning professionals are tasked with creating extra slots for training at the end of the training schedule, while earlier classes remain empty or lightly attended. The influence of organizational leaders and project sponsors can help enforce training attendance so that resources are best utilized, last-minute training is avoided, and staff are not locked out of the system at implementation due to the lack of training.

Leaders and project sponsors are also an important resource when implementing training for groups such as providers. Providers that are not employed by the organization where training is being offered have busy schedules and practices to run. Attending training classes requires the provider to cancel appointments or readjust their schedule, and the training class often falls to the lowest priority in the provider's day. Closing a private provider practice or reducing the patient schedule can impact revenue. In addition, providers with privileges at multiple organizations may be required to attend multiple classes on multiple systems, requiring even more of their time. Leaders are able to help with provider engagement and to help stress the need and importance of the training content.

Providers employed by the organization implementing HIT may face fewer barriers for attending a training class. Employed providers may not have a practice to run, or may have more latitude to adjust patient appointments and schedules during training without a large impact on revenue. For employed providers, the leadership team may choose to close a practice or cut operational hours with minimal impact to the overall organization.

When training providers, whether employed or not, learning professionals may consider offering training sessions at night and on the weekend. It may be beneficial to the provider learning audience to offer remote training sessions for those who may already be proficient in the new system from practicing at another facility. When difficulties arise with engaging provider practices or gaining training buy-in, senior organizational leaders are often able to work with provider groups and their leaders, including chiefs of staff, to develop a training solution that is satisfactory to all.

HIT training within the acute setting requires a large amount of coordination, and leaders must be supportive of a training plan that may start up to 90 days before system implementation, and involves classes around the clock. When faced with a large volume of learners to train, juggling duties that give them little available time, leaders will need to develop a plan to address staff who do not attend training. Some organizations will not provide access to a new system until training has been completed while others may provide access to the system along with at the elbow support from the trainers. Both of these options will have an impact on organizational revenue and operations.

When planning for training, space for classes may also become an issue, especially during a pandemic when learners must be distanced from each other. When classrooms must accommodate fewer people, leaders should be part of the decision to either extend the training schedule, find alternative ways to deliver training, or to locate additional training facilities. When space is limited, leaders occasionally authorize the funds to rent a hotel conference room or similar larger facility. Be aware that any off-site training solution will also require extra funds for moving and setting up equipment as well as IT support during the class time.

The Informatics Nurse as a Leader in HIT Training

The role of nursing informatics (NI) in HIT projects can vary depending on the organization. Some NI work at the executive level and in this functional level the focused is on being visionary and making sure that technology aligns with organizational goals. The NI may also work in middle management, and working at that level may involve management of all phases of an HIT project and its resources. In some situations, the NI may not have direct oversight of the people or phases of a project and must lead by influence to ensure the success of a project.

Leading by Influence

In many cases when a health care system has multiple facilities, the project team may involve members from the corporate office, and members from the individual facility. These team members often report to different leaders and may have different goals and priorities. Leading by influence means that the leader or NI involved in the project, without positional authority over other staff, needs to develop a solid working relationship with all team members. Through inclusion, open communication, and idea sharing the team can unite and perform well under a leader without direct positional authority.

To influence is to impose an impression on the performances, mindsets, attitudes, and decisions that others make, and it shouldn't resemble control in any way. Leading by influence should not use manipulation to produce results, but rather involve being aware of what motivates people to commit to a situation, and using that information to influence performance. A leader's ability to have influence is rooted in trust. To build trust, seek ideas from others, especially if they will be impacted, this demonstrates that that the leader is concerned and helps to build up trust. A leader should also exhibit passion, a leader's passion for a project will ignite others to join in to accomplish a successful project. Lastly, a leader should be open to being influenced by others, this will help to build respect and trust which ultimately increases influence. Nursing informaticists often lead people by using a natural nursing ability to get the work done. The American Nurse Association (ANA) [8] outlines and endorses the skillset of leadership for the nurse informaticist and has been doing so since informatics was identified as a specialty in 1992.

The Scope of NI Responsibility as a Leader

Training is one of the most important steps of any HIT project and it has a direct impact on the success or failure of the project. The NI can have responsibility over many different parts of HIT implementations such as obtaining funding, participating in system design, engaging end users, developing a go-live strategy, managing enhancements, developing and participating in a governance structure, creating downtime processes, evaluating the system, collecting lessons learned, and communication. Additional details of the NI responsibilities are provided below.

Obtain Funding

In both executive and middle management, NI can have the responsibility of obtaining funding for HIT projects. The responsibility can consist of grant writing to secure funds or requesting engagement with vendors to obtain quotes and proposals. Training has an impact on finance and the NI is involved in decisions about how training will be conducted such as length, location, training personnel, and staffing. Issues impacting the budget are all important components for the NI to consider when leading HIT projects.

Participate in System Design

In a middle management position, the NI can have the responsibility to participate in system design, which covers all of the phases of the System Develop Life Cycle (SDLC), which includes analysis, design, testing, training, implementation, evaluation, and maintenance. When all of the SDLC phases are performed correctly, the system design will be more efficient and effective, and more likely to be on time and on budget.

Engage End-Users

End users are those who will ultimately be using the HIT system once implemented. It is imperative that end-users are engaged in all phases of the project, because the project success depends on adoption of the technology by the end users. NIs in both executive and middle management positions are positioned to engage end-users. Executive level NIs can share the vision of the organization and how technology is needed to help achieve the goals. The middle management NI can engage the end-user by giving them a voice at the different stages of the project, enabling them to have more system ownership as part of the team.

Go-Live Strategy

In both executive and middle management positions, NIs can be instrumental in putting a strategy together for go-live. System go-lives have many working parts that have to come together minute by minute, and it takes the input of many stakeholders to achieve a solid strategy. Contrary to what some leaders may believe, a system implementation is not a plug and play process. Training the staff to use the new system is one of the most important parts of a go-live strategy, and the voice of the learning professional must be part of the strategic planning.

Enhancements

Once a system has been implemented, there will be opportunities to enhance and improve the system. About 60–120 days post go-live the end-users will understand the system more and will be able to think about how to make the system better. Every organization should have a process that outlines how enhancements to the system are to be requested and how long to wait after system implementation until changes are to be made. The NI and the learning professional should be an integral part of setting up and participating in the enhancement process. As changes are made to the system, the learning professional will need to be engaged to communicate or teach changes to the system.

Governance Structure

Both executive and middle management NI positions should have a role in developing the governance structure which is needed to maintain and enhance the system. Changes to HIT systems will be ongoing, and the governance structure will guide the team through the decision-making process while keeping the work aligned with the organizational goals. Learning professionals are impacted by the governance structures when it relates to the training that is needed when changes are made to the system. Training materials will need to stay up to date, and some organizations use tip sheets to communicate minor changes. Tip sheets can easily be sent by email and housed in a tip sheet repository.

Downtime Processes

All HIT systems will experience both planned and unplanned downtimes. Each system will have routine updates that require the system to be down for a period of time. The NI leading the HIT project will play a role in outlining the downtime process. Planned downtimes are typically done in the off hours so that routine business is disrupted the least. However, unplanned downtimes can happen at any time and staff need to be prepared for both situations. As learning professionals, it will be important to include the downtime processes in the training materials, and the processes should be covered during training, and for new hires.

Evaluate

Evaluation is imperative and can be performed by both executive and managerial level NIs. Every project implementation should be evaluated to measure success and to learn from mistakes made. Unfortunately, this step in a HIT implementation sometimes can get overlooked and can lead to poor adoption along with many other impacts. Learning professionals also provide an evaluation at the end of the training so stakeholders can understand what went well and what did not. This information is used to improve future training sessions.

Lessons Learned

The NI is involved in *lessons learned* activities. This process occurs at the completion of a project implementation when the whole project team comes together to discuss what went well and what did not. The feedback received during this activity lets the project leaders know what to change or keep for future projects.

Communicate, Communicate, and Communicate

With any project, communication is important to project success. The NI communicates with different individuals throughout the project, starting at the beginning and continuing after implementation. Because there are so many stakeholders involved in an HIT implementation project, frequent communication allows all stakeholders to be addressed. Communication can impact the success of a project, and it is very difficult to over communicate. The NI and learning professionals are knowledgeable about when to communicate, who needs communication, and the method to use to communicate with each stakeholder. The goal of communication is to get the correct information to the right people and for an HIT implementation project, the right cadence of communication to the right people is the key to a great implementation.

Summary

Leaders are a critical element for the success of an HIT project and the training plan. Leaders may not be aware of all of the details of the coming technology, nor the importance of training for the success of the project. It is important for the learning professional, often the informatics nurse, to effectively engage with leaders so that barriers to success are removed and needed resources can be secured. Engaging with leaders requires an understanding of leadership styles and communication preferences so that communication is positive and effective. When the informatics nurse is in a leadership role, they are well-positioned to facilitate the success of both HIT training and the system implementation.

Discussion Questions and Answers

1. What are some of the differences between a transactional leader and a transformational leader? As a learning professional, how would you tailor your communication when engaging with these two types of leaders?

   The transactional leader views the work of their staff as a transaction. This type of leader will reward good work with praise, a favor, an elevated standing in the organization or department, or by granting another request based on successful completion of a task. The transactional leader will also consider consequences for work that is not completed as prescribed. In this case, the leader may withdraw approval and favor, may assign a task to another person as a sign of decreasing trust, or may express their thoughts and disappointments about the perceived failure.

   The transformational leader views work as a part of the movement towards a larger goal and is appreciative of ideas and plans that further movement towards the goal. When faced with problems, the transformational leader expects to hear potential solutions for the problem and will support staff with the resources they need to reach goals. The transformational leader may also reiterate the vision to ensure that team members are still aligned and moving towards the vision.

2. What are the positive aspects of each of the five different leadership styles? If your training project is experiencing issues, how would you expect each of the five different leadership styles to help address the project issues?

   Each of the leadership styles have strong points that shine in specific situations.

   - *The transactional leader can often produce resources and additional support for a project by relying on past favors provided to others. Additionally, the staff reporting to a transactional leader are very clear about expectations and are provided real-time feedback on their work.*
   - *The transformational leader is a wonderful resource for a new project or major organizational change because they can create a vision and engage their teams to move towards that vision. The transformational leader empowers their teams to create the solutions needed to move towards the vision.*
   - *Democratic leaders prefer to involve all team members in decision-making, thus reinforcing ownership of decisions and changes. Because many people are involved in decision-making, democratic leaders are good at addressing complex issues by having the ability to bring multiple perspectives to the table.*
   - *Laissez-faire leaders do not typically micromanage their staff and therefore allow their staff a large amount of trust and latitude to devise and implement solutions to presented problems. When employees feel trusted, they often work harder and are more creative in their approaches to getting work done.*
   - *Autocratic leaders appreciate rules and policies and are very good at ensuring that processes are followed as intended and that policies are present and implemented. The autocratic leader makes quick decisions because they are solely responsible for decision-making.*

3. Imagine that your training project champion, the chief nursing officer (CNO), is an autocratic leader. The CNO is not familiar with the evidence and research supporting training methodology and is insisting that training be delivered using PowerPoint hand-outs and presentations. How would you deal with this CNO champion? Are there any other resources you could utilize when there is a major disagreement over the training project plans?

- *There are several options for dealing with a leader who has their own rigid ideas about how things should be done. There are several approaches that could be considered in the situation presented here.*
- *If you are not the leader of the project, include your leader in conversations with the CNO so that the issues are clearly understood and acknowledged.*
- *If the CNO is not interested in hearing evidence about best training approaches and insists on her way of completing the training, it may be beneficial to speak with other senior leaders who are aware of the training project. Presenting a non-biased overview of the current situation and evidence of the benefits of using a different training plan, or evidence of the harm that may occur may help other senior leaders to intervene.*
- *The ultimate goal is to influence the stance of the CNO so that they are able to understand and support a more evidence-based approach to training. To help this occur, consider involving the CNO is some problem-solving related to the project, get them involved in a training conference or seminar, or help them to remember some instances of poor training that they have had in their past and use those examples and memories to improve the current project.*

References

1. McBride S, Tietze M, Robichaux C, Stokes L, Weber E. Identifying and addressing ethical issues with use of electronic health records. Online J Issues Nurs. 2018;23(1):6–6. https://doi.org/10.3912/OJIN.
2. Ko M, Wagner L, Spetz J. Nursing home implementation of health information technology: review of the literature finds inadequate investment in preparation, infrastructure, and training. Inquiry. 2018; https://doi.org/10.1177/0046958018778902.
3. Manning J. The influence of nurse manager leadership style on staff nurse work engagement. J Nurs Adm. 2016;46:438–43. https://doi.org/10.1097/NNA.0000000000000372.
4. Schooley S (2019) What kind of leader are you? 9 leadership types and their strengths. *Business News Daily*. Retrieved December 7, 2021 from https://www.businessnewsdaily.com/9789-leadership-types.html.
5. Mackenzie S, Podsakoff P, Rich G. Transformational and transactional leadership and salesperson performance. J Acad Mark Sci. 2001;29(2):115–34. https://doi.org/10.1177/03079459994506.
6. Vesterinen S, Isola A, Paasivaara L. Leadership styles of Finnish nurse managers and factors influencing it. J Nurs Manag. 2009;17(4):503–9. https://doi.org/10.1111/j.1365-2834.2009.00989.x.

7. Merrill K. RN leadership style and patient safety. JONA: J Nurs Adm. 2015;45(6):319–24. https://doi.org/10.1097/NNA.0000000000000207.
8. American Nurses Association. (ANA, 2015) Nursing Informatics: Scope and Standards of Practice, 2nd.

Renee Robinson holds an MSN and DNP from Walden University and is board certified in nursing informatics. She is currently the director of ambulatory clinical informatics at LifeBridge Health and brings experience in designing, building, testing, training, implementing and evaluation of EHRs to her role. In addition, Dr. Robinson teaches nursing informatics at Vanderbilt University School of Nursing. Her experience as a nurse includes women's oncology, medical-surgery and cardiopulmonary care, nursing leadership, and informatics leadership. Dr. Robinson's areas of focus include optimizing ambulatory EHR workflows and governance structures.

Chapter 4
Managing Change through Training

Deborah Lewis and Brenda Kulhanek

Abstract Organizational changes occur frequently and impact the way people work. Training is an important part of the change process, and often the last exposure prior to the change comes from the training process. Because of this, training should address both the organizational and the individual's response to change, including personal and emotional factors. Learning professionals should be familiar with change theories and have the ability to incorporate evidence-based change methods into training for the best learning outcomes.

Keywords Change · Motivation · Adoption · Freeze · Communication

Progress is Impossible without Change—*Walt Disney*

Learning Outcomes
1. Define change as it relates to training
2. Discuss the use of theory to support training
3. Identify four change management theories and explain how they are used to support training
4. Describe the importance of a communication plan for training
5. Analyze the importance of change theory in evaluation of training
6. Describe strategies to support lasting change

D. Lewis
Doctoral Program, College of Nursing, Walden University, Minneapolis, MN, USA

B. Kulhanek (✉)
School of Nursing, Vanderbilt University, Nashville, TN, USA

© The Author(s), under exclusive license to Springer Nature Switzerland AG 2022
B. Kulhanek, K. Mandato (eds.), *Healthcare Technology Training*, Health Informatics, https://doi.org/10.1007/978-3-031-10322-3_4

33

The Importance of Managing Change

Change is a certainty in healthcare. Once of the biggest changes experienced by a healthcare organization is the transition from paper charting to computerized charting in the electronic health record (EHR), or from one EHR system to another. The following story is a compilation of actual events that have occurred across the globe. Imagine that an organization has selected the EHR technology that best fits the organization, investing millions of dollars in the software, technology, and staffing needed to build and implement the system. Most of the focus of the organizational leaders and the project team has been on the development of the software, and the installation of technology that will create a solid network and access to the EHR for all nurses and care providers. Unnoticed by leaders is the undercurrent of dissent about the upcoming EHR implementation. Nurses, nursing leaders, physicians, and other caregivers have only been told that the EHR will be implemented in the near future. Nurses with minimal computer experience are anxious and afraid that they will no longer be able to do their work, and physicians are worried about the time that this new system will take away from their daily practice. As tensions mount, a few of the more vocal staff begin to emerge as leaders of an EHR opposition group.

Five weeks before the EHR is to be implemented, staff started their training classes to learn to use the new system. Training was focused only on the functionality of the new system and there was no opportunity during training for staff to express concerns or to learn more about how other organizations had successfully implemented this same system. Finally, the big day arrived. Nurses were required to carry their full patient load as they started to use this new computer system. No paper charts were available for reference and patient care suffered for weeks as nurses struggled to locate information in the EHR and document in the correct location. Over time, more and more staff started aligning with the most vocal opponents of the new EHR system. The number of nurses calling out sick increased daily, and a growing number of nurses were turning in their resignations. Some providers started sending their patients to competitor hospitals in protest of the new EHR system. Faced with unhappy staff, declining admissions, and physician opposition, the surprised hospital leaders made the decision to discontinue implementation of the new EHR system and revert back to paper charts. How did this multi-million-dollar implementation become derailed?

Defining Change

Change is a dynamic and ongoing process in most organizations. Change impacts the way people work; their duties, the scope of their responsibilities and who they report to and interact with. These changes cause anxiety and can be alleviated by transparency about the overall organizational and individual impacts of the change. Training is one component of the change process, and often the last exposure to the new technology and processes before the change will occur. Because of this, training should be prepared to address both the organizational and the individual's response to change, including personal and emotional factors. Organizational change is ongoing and effective training must be designed to support both the human and organizational responses to change.

The motivation to change is based in part on previous experiences with change. There are a number of personal and emotional factors that can influence change. These factors must be considered when planning training:

Individual

How will change impact the work, role, and reporting relationship for each individual? Will the change impact job security?

Organization

How will the organization be impacted by this change? Will the organization remain viable? How will the organization's mission and vision change?

Customer

How will consumers be impacted by this change? What will this change mean for the community and the patients? The change management models and theories presented in this chapter will help to address the impact of change for the individual, organization, and customer.

A Change in Knowledge Versus a Change in Behavior

Training is about individuals' acceptance of new initiatives that result in practice changes. Some individuals and institutions may readily accept new ideas, yet resist changes in behaviors. Attitudes have long been recognized as important predictors of individual differences in educational application, learning and achievement. It is important to consider how new initiatives or practice changes can be shared with individuals in a way that is informative, engaging and motivating. Positive acceptance of new initiatives and practice changes is the goal, and the way that training is designed can facilitate a more rapid acceptance of change, and support a positive transformation.

When supporting change through training it is important to align the training with the organization's mission and vision. Organizational leadership must be committed to providing needed resources that support the plan for training.

Senior level individuals in an organization are necessary to help plan and support training. It is also important to set the stage for peer-to-peer training and include conversations that provide stories of success related to the change to support individuals' readiness for change.

Change is supported when a shift of responsibility from the trainer to the learner occurs. Well-designed training acknowledges potential resistance to change. If change has not been addressed, a struggle to accept training may exist resulting in decreased effectiveness of training methods, and minimal knowledge acquisition.

Finally, it is important to ensure that training is easy to understand and applicable to the individual's role. If possible and appropriate, it is advisable to provide opportunities to practice and reinforce the training as a way to manage the anxiety produced by change.

Using Theory to Support Training

Once it has been determined that training is the appropriate intervention, learning theories and models should be considered during the development phase to inform the design of the training program. By envisioning the training topic from different theoretical perspectives, learning professionals can best understand how to deliver new information that helps to fill gaps in knowledge while also supporting motivation, engagement, and the desired change. Change theory provides a framework and the foundational assumptions that support the development of the training program. Figure 4.1 depicts the flow of theory-based training that incorporates motivation and engagement to support knowledge and behavior change.

Fig. 4.1 Theory-based training

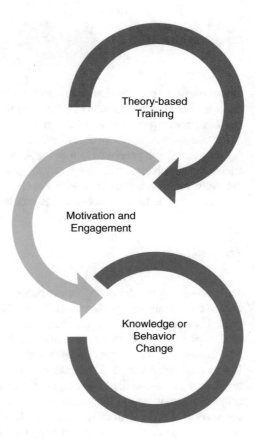

Change Management Theories

Change occurs in every healthcare setting; it is part of the processes that support ongoing organizational and practice growth. Change theorists have provided multiple approaches for facilitating change in an organization and within an individual experiencing change. Change theories and models provide a foundation for understanding the response to change, guiding successful change, and designing training and communication to best support successful change.

Lewin's Change Theory

Kurt Lewin, one of the leading psychologists of his time, introduced the three-step model of change. The three steps model has long served as a fundamental approach to organizational/ behavioral change (Fig. 4.2). The model outlines steps that include unfreezing, moving, and refreezing [1]. Lewin detailed change as an

Fig. 4.2 Kurt Lewin—
changing as three steps

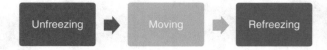

alteration of a force field that represents the current state, and proposed that the change agent or trainer needs to think in terms of how the existing training environment is transformed into a desired state for change. Seeing social habits as inner resistance to change, Lewin described that a successful change includes three stages: (1) unfreezing the present, (2) moving forward with change, and (3) refreezing or anchoring the change. Success at any stage is determined by a level of adoption by the individuals involved [2]. Therefore, changing the attitudes or behaviors of individuals is central to the success of Lewin's model [3].

Unfreezing

The first step of the three-step model begins with unfreezing of the present practice or ways of doing things. Lewin believed that human behavior was based on the preference of individuals to maintain a sense of equilibrium. He described the need to disrupt or unfreeze that equilibrium so that old notions could be unlearned and new behaviors and changes could be adopted [4]. In order to achieve unfreezing, Lewin contended that it is necessary to guide the individual to a deliberate emotional transformation [2]. Lewin equated this concept with Gordon Allport's description of catharsis where the individual must first deal with the existing emotional connection to bring about change [5]. In the unfreezing stage the individual may be unaware of the need for change and may not be ready to accept change. Planning for training occurs at this stage and should include a supportive message to all individuals regarding the upcoming change. Sharing data and evidence to support the change should also be incorporated into the initial message.

Moving

The second stage of moving is when the change actually occurs and is underway [3]. Lewin referred to moving as a form of motion or shift that occurs when "the forces pressing for change are greater than those resisting change" ([1] p. 50). This stage occurs as the organization moves or transitions to the new change and involves the delivery of the training module or program. Lewin described the notion of driving forces or the forces that can help to drive the change. This is an important concept to consider during the moving phase, and these driving forces should include individual champions who can help to motivate and support the change [6].

Refreezing

The third and final stage of Lewin's three steps model is refreezing. Refreezing occurs when training is completed and is also the time when new organizational policies and practices are formalized and launched. This stage suggests that the change has been adopted. Refreezing seeks to maintain stability or the new equilibrium of the change, reducing the opportunity for regression [4]. For refreezing to be sustained the change in practice or new ideas must be in congruence with the behavior, personality, and environment of the individual or it may lead to ongoing resistance [7]. Lewin believed that one means of bringing about change in individuals was through positive group support [3]. If group norms are transformed and new changes are adopted at the group level then individual behavior can be sustained [1]. Champions for change and organization leaders need to share key outcomes of the new initiatives with all involved.

Rogers' Diffusion of Innovation

Everett Rogers studied the process of adoption of change, or innovation, by the individual in an organization. The diffusion of innovation and new ideas occurs through information that is communicated by individuals through a communication network or social system [8–10]. Diffusion is specifically defined by Rogers as a way to communicate or spread messages perceived as dealing with new ideas, while also representing a certain degree of uncertainty for an individual or organization [11].

Innovations represent new ideas and practice changes that are related to a gap in a participant's current practice and lead toward development of new goals. Diffusion is the process through which innovations are communicated and adopted. Prior conditions influence the decision to adopt, these may include the individuals understanding of the need for change, level of agreement with innovations or change, adherence to old norms, and prior ways of practice. The adoption of an innovation often proceeds in stages that may or may not be sequential. Rogers [10] identified the stages of diffusion of innovation as knowledge, persuasion, decision, implementation, and confirmation (Table 4.1).

Innovations are commonly adopted by way of organizational communication channels. This can be supported during training when individuals observe the behavior of trusted opinion leaders [12]. Innovation adopters, or change adopters, can be characterized as ranging from innovators, early adopters, early majority, late majority, and laggards [13], as illustrated in Table 4.2.

Table 4.1 Diffusion of innovation

Stage	Description
Knowledge	Awareness of the individuals, these may be socioeconomic or personal. Understanding the need for change. Communication regarding the change is key.
Persuasion	In this stage the individual person a favorable or unfavorable opinion of the change. Training needs to take into account several key components of this stage, these factors can support the rate of adoption of the proposed change: Relative advantage – The underlying motivation for individuals to perceive the change as advantageous. This motivation may be social or economic [9]. Compatibility – the individual perception that the change is consistent with the existing values, past experiences, and needs of the individual and organization [9]. Complexity – How is the change understood by the individual, change that is perceived to be complex may be adopted more slowly [9]. Trialability - The degree to which the change may be practiced or tried out. Providing practice opportunities as part of training, can support adoption of the change [9]. Observability – Making the results of the change visible to others. Supporting the effective communication of the change through trusted organizational opinion leaders [9].
Decision	In this stage individuals will most likely be engaged in training. The training and the support of opinion leaders can support their decision to adopt the change or reject the change.
Implementation	Training is completed and the individuals and organization are implementing the change. Some individuals may still be considering adoption of the change.
Confirmation	Individuals and organizations evaluate the results of the change. For the individuals the evaluation may include personal and social impacts.

Table 4.2 Innovation adoption characteristics

Stage	Standard deviation	Description
Innovators		Innovators are the individuals willing to take risks. They will be eager to adopt and share the change with others. They can be opinion leaders to help facilitate change.
Early adopters		Early adopters want to understand the change and are willing to participate in training. They can be important individuals in planning for change and are important opinion leaders to communicate the change [8].
Early majority		Early majority adopt a change after innovators and early adopters. Adoption for this group may happen after training has occurred [8].
Late majority		Late majority have a degree of skepticism and may take a longer time to adopt the change.
Laggards		Laggards are the last to adopt an innovation, they usually resist and may never adopt the change [8].

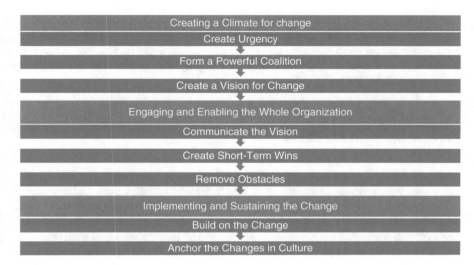

Fig. 4.3 The 8-step model

Kotter's 8-Step Model for Change

John Kotter [14] introduced his eight-step change process to promote organizational change (Fig. 4.3). Kotter's approach is a proven method to implement systemic change by providing a roadmap which highlights principals to achieve transformational change [15]. According to Kotter, management serves as a set of processes for keeping a given system functioning well or keeping some activity under control [16]. Kotter's theory of change has demonstrated beneficial effects across multi-organizational stages of management [17].

As expressed in Kotter's change management philosophy, change has both emotional and situational components that are detailed in his 8-step model. Each of these steps can be divided into 3 phases: (1) creating a climate for change, (2) engaging and enabling the whole organization, (3) implementing and sustaining the change [14].

Creating a Climate for Change

Create Urgency

In step one, the establishment of a sense of urgency entails identifying any threats or repercussions that have the potential to appear that in turn enables the need to achieve change. If people do not see the need, they will not change [18]. Urgency can force the examination of opportunities that are unlocked through intervention or discussion. Then, additional support or engagement from the appropriate individuals such as subject matter experts can be requested in order to facilitate change. By addressing the problem, positive and sustainable change can be fostered. This first step motivates the group to support change by highlighting the need to resolve a key issue or problem [19].

Form a Powerful Coalition

To create a guiding coalition, the assembly of committed leaders and/or stakeholders within organizations is necessary to lead the desired change [18]. Collaboration will ensure the involvement and engagement from cross-functional areas and departments contributes to the formulation of a powerful and diverse coalition. In this context, a guiding coalition includes respected leaders who can motivate and encourage others to adopt new ideas or practice changes [19].

Create a Vision for Change

Creating a vision and grand strategy for change helps to outline what kind of change is needed and how it can be actualized. Through this development, change can be clearly and effectively communicated by leaders in a manner that people can understand [18]. The guiding vision subsequently aids not only by steering the change but also developing strategic initiatives to achieve the specified vision [19].

Communicate the Vision

Communicating the vision of change must be done powerfully and convincingly, with clarity in the why, what, and how [18]. Once the vision for change is established, the message should be shared with individuals who are involved with planning for the change, individual and group concerns should be handled with honesty and transparency [19].

Remove Obstacles and Act on the Vision

Although a vision may be effectively communicated, the adoption of change necessitates broad-based support of change [18]. To accomplish this step, all members must endorse the vision and change while actively supporting the process to achieve it [19].

Create Short-Term Wins

By creating short-term wins at the beginning stages of the change process, then others can see how the change progresses. It is important to create many short-term targets instead of one long-term goal, which are achievable and less expensive and have lesser possibilities of failure. Reward the contributions of people who are involved in meeting the targets. Changes are easy to envision and initiate but difficult to sustain [19].

Build on the Change

To capitalize on gains and generate more change, facilitate continuous improvement by building on successes. This encourages individuals of the change and garners more sustainable support towards the vision. In this way, change will be reinforced, while the overall vision remains the central point of focus [19].

Anchor the Changes in the Culture

As a part of more long-term success, discussion of success assures others of the change and instills it as part of the organizational culture and transforms it into the norm [18].

The Human Response to Change

Kubler-Ross Change Theory

The normal human response to change involves emotions, and along with the changes in processes, the introduction of new technology elicits an emotional response for those experiencing change [20]. Although the Kubler-Ross model was first developed to address emotions seen in patients and families during the dying process, the same cycle of emotions has been noted in other circumstances and the emotional curve very closely aligns with the responses to change noted in other change theories (Table 4.3).

When a major change is first introduced, those who will be impacted by change may experience anxiety, apprehension, but also enthusiasm and motivation. As the change is implemented and the impact of the change is realized, people may exhibit depression, frustration, and a feeling of loss. Over a period of time the emotions of anger, activism, criticism of the change, and speaking out against the change may be

Table 4.3 Emotions and the change curve

Emotion	Reaction	Coping strategy
Denial	This system is riddled with so many problems, it will never be implemented	Maintain a clear message that is aligned with the organizational strategy
Anger	We had no say in which system was selected or how this system works	Identify your champions and magnify positive messages, allow time for emotions to be heard
Bargaining	We might be able to use this system if we can continue to have shadow charts or paper spreadsheets	Emphasize how training will ensure that people can use the system and be successful
Depression	This system is impossible to use and is negatively impacting my ability to care for patients or do my job	Allow for question and answer sessions, reassure the learners
Acceptance	It looks like this change is here to stay, even though it is not perfect	Realize that some will accept the change earlier than others and reward the positive attitudes
Commitment	Now that I have used the system for a while, it does have some benefits	Encourage positive attitudes and behaviors, enable peer support of others

seen among those experiencing the change. The third stage of bargaining may be seen as the anger fades into resignation. Bargaining may be seen in attempts to manipulate the change. Finally, acceptance of the change emerges along with the realization that life has changed, and perhaps the people impacted by the change have also grown and changed [21].

The Kubler-Ross change model, as in other change models, notes that the people undergoing change will not arrive at the same stages of change at the same time [22]. Although there is disagreement on the value of the Kubler-Ross change model, the emotions of those undergoing change must be recognized and incorporated into a change strategy.

Prochaska's Transtheoretical Model

The transtheoretical model of behavior change was first developed by James Prochaska as a model of intentional change that concentrates on individual decision making (Fig. 4.4). The model suggests that health behavior change involves six stages: Precontemplation, Contemplation, Determination, Action, Maintenance, Relapse [23]. In this model, behavior change is a process and individuals decide how and when they are ready to change. One factor that supports the individual's decision to accept or move to change are their perceptions of positive outcomes associated with the change. Understanding this model may help trainers design motivational elements into the training plan to support action on the part of individual learners [24, 25].

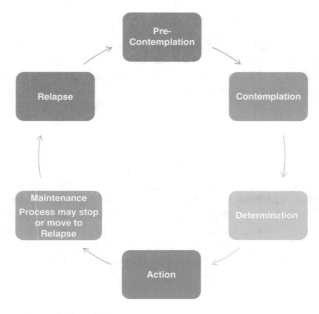

Fig. 4.4 The transtheoretical model

Six Stages of Change

Precontemplation

In this stage the individual has not acknowledged that there is a need to change or does not intend to change. This behavior can be due to resistance to change or lack of understanding of the change [26].

Contemplation

Individuals in this stage acknowledge that the change is important, and they are considering the change, but may still have mixed feelings. Motivation is important at this stage, and this is an appropriate time to provide additional information about the importance of the change. It is also a good time to engage opinion leaders and change champions to support the importance of the change. Individuals may acknowledge that there is a problem but are not yet ready or sure if they want to make a change. Contemplation involves recognition of the problem, initial consideration of behavior changes, and information gathering about possible solutions and actions.

Preparation

Individuals in this stage plan to change in the near future [26]. It is important to provide a realistic training plan that incorporates transparency especially when discussing organizational change, the personal impact, and any incentives. Preparation is also the stage where training begins.

Action

At this stage, training has occurred or is nearing completion. Individuals may have already integrated the training and made the needed changes. Individual commitment to change is important to support success at this stage [26]. Although individuals all attend similar or the same training, they still need to take individual steps for successful engagement and integration of the training received. It is important to note any individual differences and reassure the participants. During the action stage, it is a good time to provide additional support from the opinion leaders or champions.

Maintenance

This stage is about supporting and maintaining the change. Individuals have participated in the training and have experienced the resulting change for 6 months or more. It is possible that individuals who were resistant to change might fall back to old habits. Consistent support to maintain the change is important [26].

Relapse

This stage is not always included but should be acknowledged. It is possible for individuals to return to prior behaviors. When implementing a training strategy, it is important to consider a plan for ongoing monitoring and reinforcement after the initial training has been completed.

Change Communication

Regardless of the change model that is used to guide change, a communication plan will be essential for ensuring that those undergoing change have all of the information that they need to manage the change. Communication is more than speaking, writing, or disseminating a message to a person or audience. Communication must also be received and understood by the recipient to be effective.

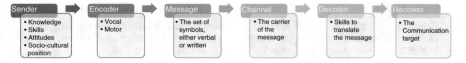

Fig. 4.5   Berlo communication model

In the 1960s a communication model was developed to document the communication process and points in the process where communication could experience disruption [27]. In the Berlo communication model (Fig. 4.5), a message consists of a sender, the message is encoded using the nuances of vocal language or writing, symbols are used in the content of the message, a channel is used to send the message, the recipient of the message must have the skills to decode the message, and the message must reach the receiver or target of the communication [28]. Communication can experience challenges in both the channel and decoding stages, when noise is experienced [29]. Issues with the channel element of the communication process can be related to lack of understanding of the communication channel, unawareness of the channel, or an inability to access the channel. In the decoding phase, noise can be caused by language, cultural, and symbolic issues within the message.

An effective communication plan will incorporate all of the elements of communication so that the message intended by the sender is clearly received by the recipient. Identified causes of communication barriers include using terms that are unfamiliar to people, anxiety, and using slang or words not commonly understood. When engaged in verbal communication, barriers can include volume of the speaker, noise, and environmental distractions such as temperature of the room [30].

Communication Tips

Content

The content for written communication should be limited whenever possible to key message elements. When sending communication in an email, the message should be no more than one paragraph and ideally formatted with the key information in bullet points for quick visual recognition and reading of the key information. Avoid images that are not necessary and leave plenty of white space around the message so that viewer can focus in on the key points (Fig. 4.6).

For verbal communication, a recorded video or audio message should be less than 2 min. If the communication is face to face, the upper limits of the adult attention space is about 20 minutes. When speaking, make sure that verbal tone is engaging with plenty of variation in inflection and tone. Volume should not be too loud or too soft for the audience to hear.

Dear colleagues:

Guided by our mission, we are focused on improving patient safety and supporting high quality patient care. To further our mission, we will be implementing an electronic health record (EHR) later this year. Benefits of the EHR will include:

- Electronic communication
- The ability for multiple people to access the patient chart from multiple locations
- Embedded evidence to guide practice
- Real-time documentation of patient care

Town hall meetings will be scheduled at various times over the next three weeks to allow for more discussion and information sharing.

-Your Leadership Team

Fig. 4.6 Concise communication

Method Effective communication that reaches the largest audience will be delivered in multiple ways. Options for sending a message will depend on the culture and practices of an organization. Some organizations have established expectations for communication while others have not. In some cases, an email message will not be an effective tool while in other cases the expectation is that email should be read frequently. Options for sending messages include email, printed messages displayed where staff gather, verbal messages, messages ingrained into shift reports, messages on electronic announcement screens, text messages, and one on one conversations. One tried and true method is to place printed communication into bathroom stalls where staff are sure to see the information!

Audience Communication should be focused on the specific audience for which the communication applies. When communication is sent to the wrong audience it can create dissatisfaction or trigger a flood of unnecessary communication. Additionally, communication should be tailored to the communication styles and preferences of the audience. If the recipient group for the communication does not have computer access, then sending an email message would not be appropriate. If communication is being sent to organizational leaders, the content of the message should be different than that sent to care providers in an organization. Typically, leaders prefer communication in the format of an executive summary, without the detail that may be necessary for other audiences.

Timing It is important to determine the purpose of a communication and time the information accordingly. For example, if the purpose of a message is for nurses to sign up for a training course time slot, the message would need to be send early enough to accommodate the staffing schedule. Detailed messages about an upcoming change in an EHR system, if sent too early, will be long forgotten by the time the changes occur.

Reinforcement The socio-cultural status of the communication sender can impact reception of the message. To reinforce communication and add gravity to the mes-

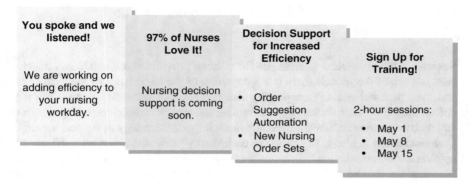

You spoke and we listened!

We are working on adding efficiency to your nursing workday.

97% of Nurses Love It!

Nursing decision support is coming soon.

Decision Support for Increased Efficiency

- Order Suggestion Automation
- New Nursing Order Sets

Sign Up for Training!

2-hour sessions:

- May 1
- May 8
- May 15

Fig. 4.7 Progressive communication

sage, it can be helpful to enlist leaders in an organization to either send communication or to reinforce a message through follow-up. Additionally, ongoing reminders and communication updates can help the retention of information. A layered approach to communication can increase interest by using curiosity to your advantage (Fig. 4.7).

Evaluation

Just as organizations change over time, communication pathways may also lose effectiveness and need to change. Periodic evaluations of communication successes and challenges can help to keep a communication plan on target. Evaluation methods for communication may be measured by viewing the number of people that access electronic communication, enlisting the assistance of unit leaders to disseminate information, or conducting spot surveys to determine if staff are aware of recent key messages.

Communication that Works

The world of healthcare is complex and can be unpredictable and chaotic. Communication that is predictable can be the difference between effective communication and ignored communication. When staff learn to expect to see a newsletter, email, or message on a certain day or at a certain time, they are more likely to make the effort to view and absorb the information. When creating a communication process and cadence, involving leaders in the development of the process will ensure their support in the ongoing communication process.

Creating a Climate for Change: Reinforcing Change during Training

Reviewing the theoretical foundations for training provides some notable consistencies. In each of the models there is a recognition of the importance of the individual and their personal goals. Transparency and provision of information regarding the change are important to set the stage for training and acceptance of change. Engagement and motivation are described universally as an important strategy to support training. Communication is also a key factor in each theory presented along with the use of opinion leaders and change champions to engage participants in support for the change. Planning for change with organizational leaders to ensure buy-in and considering ongoing training to support long-term engagement is also noted across theories. Some specific examples for how theory can be used to support training are described below.

Adoption of Innovation

Diffusion of new ideas and innovation depends in part on the training being viewed as in harmony with the goals of the individual learners and the organization. Exploration of the factors related to adoption of new ideas is an important first step in the process of change. When planning training it is important to identify the driving and restraining forces for the proposed change. One of those driving forces can be the engagement of what Rogers [10] calls early adopters. Individual adoption of innovation is described on a continuum from innovators to early adopters to laggards or those who resist or never adopt the change. Engaging innovators who are eager for the change to occur and early adopters who are motivated to learn and engage in the change process can support training success. These individuals can provide encouragement and support to their peers and can serve as champions or opinion leaders for the change.

Fun Theory

While it was not described as a stand-alone theory, the use of fun and humor can support training. Using fun in the design of training can increase engagement and reduce resistance. Fun can be applied in the form of gamification or as motivational incentives. Dalton [31] created a piano keyboard on a staircase as a way to motivate people to take the stairs. The social experiment resulted in 61% more individuals using the stairs, changing their behavior through a fun activity.

Oestreich et al. [32] conducted a qualitative analysis of graduate students' perception of the use of an escape room designed to introduce them to the process of grant submission. Their analysis identified common themes of excitement (63%), fun (50%), stress (38%), and frustration (25%). Sixty-three percent of learners preferred the escape room to didactic learning and found it beneficial to learning. Game-based learning is described by Chua [33] as an important strategy to make training applicable, meaningful, memorable, and fun for your participants. He also notes that when training is delivered with passion the learners are more engaged.

Kotter's Theory in Practice

The eight steps of Kotter's theory can be applied to training in many ways, here is one example related to organization change and training:

- **Highlight the Urgency**: Identify the reasons for the change, and why is it important. Note any internal or external factor that may be sparking the change. Aziz [34] presents the use of Kotter's eight steps to prevent needle stick injuries in a healthcare organization. In the first step staff were made aware of the problem by sharing the data regarding the number of healthcare workers who had experienced workplace needle stick injuries. They also shared the personal story of the impact of needle stick injuries on individuals and the financial impact on the organization from needle stick injuries.
- **Build the Team**: Identify the team that will implement the change. Who will lead the change? In this stage it is important to build a team that will encourage buy-in for the change. Senior staff and leadership need to be aligned to ensure that the goal of reducing workplace needle sticks is in the hands of the right team.
- **Create the Vision for Change**: How will things be in the future? The team needs to identify the potential benefits for healthcare workers and the organization that will arise, including a safer work environment.
- **Share the New Vision**: Have meetings with staff to explain the need for change and to gain insights into the staff's perspective. Following this step will encourage engagement and set the stage for the change.
- **Empower Action**: Peers and training champions should have additional transparent conversations with individuals to share information regarding the need for the upcoming training program to reduce needle stick injuries. Attempt to understand individual concerns so they may be incorporated into the training program.
- **Create Quick Wins**: Establish training goals that will ensure understanding of the training program to reduce needle stick injuries. Provide quick training that is designed to fit with the flow of the unit that is accompanied by introduction of new safety shield needles
- **Track the Progress**: Evaluate the individuals' understanding of the new safety devices. Track the incidence of needle stick injuries. Share successes and evaluate issues.
- **Strengthen the Change**: Consider any revisions to training indicated by the evaluation, revise training if needed and integrate the new safety devices to reduce needle stick injuries in the new organization.

Making Change Last

Why Does Change Fail?

Change takes time, and when shortcuts are taken that eliminate some of the steps needed for long-lasting change, the change is more likely to experience problems and failure in the future. Causes for change failure include presenting a weak sense of urgency, the absence or poor visibility of a guiding alliance of change leaders, an unclear or missing vision, poor and infrequent communication, obstacles that block change progress, failure to celebrate achievement of goals, early declaration of change success, and a corporate culture that is not embedded into the change [35].

How to Keep Change Going

Once a change has been implemented, it is important to maintain a focus on the change to ensure that newly acquired skills and processes do not degrade or disappear. Sustained change should be viewed as the responsibility of not only the training team, but also organizational leaders. Factors to consider for sustaining change include a training model for new hires who enter an organization after the initial change, identification of audit tools and reports that provide insight into the success of the change on daily work, the development of written workflow processes that can be used as an ongoing reference tool, and integration of the change into the daily work and culture of the organization [36].

Summary

Change within an organization involves a carefully designed change plan, effective communication, the support of leaders, alignment with organizational strategy, and integration into the culture of an organization. Change is supported by effective and timely communication, and through the impact of an organizational culture. Training is often the final event before a change is implemented, underscoring the importance of embedding change strategies and enablers into the training program as well as the communication regarding change. Facilitating successful change is not the responsibility of one person or team, but requires the involvement of many different stakeholders within an organization to develop and deliver successful change strategies.

Discussion Questions and Answers
1. What are the three categories of personal and emotional factors that must be considered when planning training?

- Personal: how will I be impacted by this change? how will my role change? who will I report to after the change? will I still have a job after this change?
- Organizational: how will the organization be impacted by this change? Will the organization be sustainable, how will our mission and vision change?
- Consumers (patients): how will our consumers be impacted by this change? What will change mean for our community? What will change mean for our patients?

2. Why is a change in knowledge not the end goal of training?

   - The goal of training is to change behavior, learners need knowledge to understand and implement the changes in behavior

3. Describe how you have seen the Diffusion of Innovation theory in your organization.

   - Encourage participants to share stories of changes they have experienced, ask them to identify how the diffusion of innovation theory was seen within their stories

4. What are some ways to work with "laggards" to ensure the success of a change?

   - Identify your potential laggards, engage them in the change project, seek to make your laggards your champions, take time to give the laggards a clear picture of the change to alleviate anxiety and resistance

5. At what point in the Berlo communication model can communication be disrupted and why does this happen?

   - The point where communication is most prone to disruption is between the carrier of the message and decoding the message. This can happen when the wrong carrier is selected for a message, such as using email for communication in a department where nurses never check their email. Decoding a message can be disrupted if the message is not concise and clear, if the message is never viewed, or is not targeted to the recipient audience

References

1. Burnes B. The origins of Lewin's three-step model of change. J Appl Behav Sci. 2019;56(1):32–59. https://doi.org/10.1177/0021886319892685.
2. Lewin K. Frontiers in group dynamics. Hum Relat. 1947;1(2):143–53. https://doi.org/10.1177/001872674700100201.
3. Burnes B, Bargal D. Kurt Lewin: 70 years on. J Chang Manag. 2017;17(2):91–100. https://doi.org/10.1080/14697017.2017.1299371.
4. Burnes B. Kurt Lewin and the planned approach to change: a re-appraisal. J Manag Stud. 2004;41(6):977–1002. https://doi.org/10.1111/j.1467-6486.2004.00463.x.
5. Allport GW. Catharis and the reduction of prejudice. J Soc Issues. 1945;1(3):3–10. https://doi.org/10.1111/j.1540-4560.1945.tb02687.x.

6. Cummings S, Bridgman T, Brown KG. Unfreezing change as three steps: rethinking Kurt Lewin's legacy for change management. Hum Relat. 2016;69(1):33–60.
7. Schein EH. Kurt Lewin's change theory in the field and in the classroom: notes toward a model of managed learning. Syst Pract. 1996;9(1):27–47. https://doi.org/10.1007/bf02173417.
8. Rogers EM. Diffusion of innovations. 1st ed. Free Press; 1962.
9. Rogers EM. Diffusion of innovations. 3rd ed. Free Press; 1995.
10. Rogers EM. Diffusion of innovations. 5th ed. Free Press; 2003.
11. Rogers EM. Diffusion of preventive innovations. Addict Behav. 2002;27(6):989–93. https://doi.org/10.1016/s0306-4603(02)00300-3.
12. Singhal A, Dearing JW. Communication of innovations. A journey with Everett Rogers. Am J Prev Med. 2006;31:4S.
13. Dearing JW, Cox JG. Diffusion of innovations theory, principles, and practice. Health Aff. 2018;37(2):183–90. https://doi.org/10.1377/hlthaff.2017.1104.
14. Kotter JP. Leading change. Harvard Business School Press; 1996.
15. Thornton B, Usinger J, Sanchez J. Leading effective building level change. Education. 2019;139(3):131–8.
16. Kotter JP. Leading change: a conversation with John P. Kotter. Strateg Leadersh. 1997;25(1):18–23. https://doi.org/10.1108/eb054576.
17. Maclean DFW, Vannet N. Improving trauma imaging in Wales through Kotter's theory of change. Clin Radiol. 2016;71(5):4.
18. Appelbaum SH, Habashy S, Malo JL, Shafiq H. Back to the future: revisiting Kotter's 1996 change model. J Manag Dev. 2012;31(8):764–82. https://doi.org/10.1108/02621711211253231.
19. Small A, Gist D, Souza D, Dalton J, Magny-Normilus C, David D. Using Kotter's change model for implementing bedside handoff. J Nurs Care Qual. 2016;31(4):304–9. https://doi.org/10.1097/ncq.0000000000000212.
20. Firoozmand N. Managing resistance to change. Train J. 2014:27–31.
21. Elrod PD, Tippett DD. The "death valley" of change. J Organ Chang Manag. 2002;15(3):273–91.
22. O'Shea T (2014). The Emotions of Change: Based on the Kubler-Ross Change Curve. Retrieved July 12, 2022 from https://www.hr.com/en/magazines/personal_excellence_essentials/septemer_2014_personal/the-emotions-of-change-based-on-the-kubler-ross-ch_i280ai7s.html.
23. Prochaska JO. Systems of psychotherapy: a transtheoretical analysis. Dorsey; 1979.
24. Prochaska JO, Norcross JC, DiClemente CC. Changing for good. Morrow; 1994.
25. Prochaska JO, Prochaska JO. Behavior change. In: Nash DB, Reifsnyder R, Fabius J, Pracilio VP, editors. Population health: creating a culture of wellness. Jones & Bartlett Learning; 2011. p. 23–39.
26. Lach H, Everard K, Highstein G, Brownson C. Application of the trans-theoretical model to health education for older adults. Health Promot Pract. 2004;5(1):88–93.
27. Berlo DK, Lemert JB, Mertz RJ. Dimensions for evaluating the acceptability of message sources. Public Opin Q. 1970;33(4):563–76. https://doi.org/10.1086/267745.
28. Stead BA. Berlo's communication process model as applied to the behavioral theories of Maslow, Herzberg, and McGregor. Acad Manag J. 1972;15(3):389–94. https://doi.org/10.2307/254868.
29. Lee D (1988). Developing effective communications. University of Missouri-Columbia: Communications. https://mospace.umsystem.edu/xmlui/bitstream/handle/10355/50292/cm0109-1988.pdf?sequence=1&isAllowed=y
30. Jelani F, & Nordin NS (2019) Barriers to effective communication in the workplace. Retrieved February 13, 2022 from https://scholar.archive.org/search?q=Jelani+%26+Nordin+%28201 9%29&filter_time=since_2000&sort_order=time_asc
31. Dalton A. Fun for a change. Stanf Soc Innov Rev. 2010;8(2):63–4.
32. Oestreich JH, Hunt B, Cain J. Grant deadline: an escape room to simulate grant submissions. Curr Pharm Teach Learn. 2021;13(7):848–54.
33. Chua M. Making training FUN. Armed Forces Comptroller. 2017;62(4):32–4.

34. Aziz AM. A change management approach to improving safety and preventing needle stick injuries. J Infect Prev. 2017;18(5):257–62.
35. Kotter JP. Leading change: why transformation efforts fail. Harvard Business Review; 1995.
36. Silver SA, McQuillan R, Harel Z, Weizman AV, Thomas A, Nesrallah G, Bell C, Chan CT, Chertow GM. How to sustain change and support continuous quality improvement. Clin J Am Soc Nephrol. 2016;11(5):916–24.

Deborah Lewis Over the course of my faculty career, I have had extensive on-campus and online teaching experience in both undergraduate and graduate programs. I have had experience in building new nursing informatics programs as a faculty developer, member of the leadership team and as an external consultant. In my current role, I have provided coordination, teaching and leadership to online BSN, MSN, DNP and PhD in Nursing programs. My current role has also included faculty development, faculty mentorship and program evaluation. My scholarship has included NIH grant funding and publications and presentations in consumer health and chronic illness.

Brenda Kulhanek is an associate professor at the Vanderbilt University School of Nursing and has a history of leadership in both informatics and clinical education. Dr. Kulhanek holds a PhD from Capella University and a doctor of nursing practice (DNP) from Walden University. She is board certified in nursing informatics, nursing professional development, and executive leadership. Her publications include informatics textbook chapters and multiple informatics articles. She recently participated in the Scope & Standards for Nursing Informatics publication. She teaches informatics at the master's and doctoral levels and has a particular interest in strengthening nursing through nursing informatics education, and the integration of informatics into practice to support improvement of patient outcomes.

Chapter 5
Using Learning Theory and Brain Science to Guide Training

Brenda Kulhanek

Abstract Learning theories guide how training is designed, developed, and evaluated. Using learning theories to direct training design results in improved learning and training outcomes. As science has advanced, new learning theories have emerged as it is now possible to view the brain during the learning process. This chapter will review recent research that can help learning professionals identify precision-training methods that can produce the best learning outcomes.

Keywords Brain science · Cognitivism · Behaviorism · Social learning theory Humanism · Constructivism · Andragogy · Learning styles

Learning Objectives
1. Evaluate the relationship between learning theories and HIT training
2. Discuss evidence and training best practices from neuroscience
3. Identify evidence from learning science and how it applies to specific training needs
4. Discuss the difference between learning styles and learning preferences

B. Kulhanek (✉)
School of Nursing, Vanderbilt University, Nashville, TN, USA

B. Kulhanek, K. Mandato (eds.), *Healthcare Technology Training*, Health
Informatics, https://doi.org/10.1007/978-3-031-10322-3_5

The Use of Learning Theory in Training Design

John needed to create some eLearning to teach nurses how to use a new order entry function that was being added to the EHR. He remembered hearing that people may have one of four different learning styles and that training should be designed to meet the needs of all of these different types of learners. John recalled that the four learning styles included (1) people who like to see images and videos to help their learning, (2) those who like to hear narration, (3) those who learn best by reading or writing down information, and (4) those who absorb new knowledge through hands-on activities.

Within the eLearning module, John planned to include both written text and an accompanying voice-over to speak the written words. He felt that this training design approach would address two of the four learning styles. Next, John pondered about how to include the learning needs for those who like to read and write, and those who need hands-on activities to learn. After some thought, John decided that the new eLearning module would include sections where the learner would need to enter information after reading a question or case study. This approach would address the learning needs for those who prefer to read and write to learn. Finally, John included activity in the eLearning module by creating a requirement for the learner to click an arrow to move from screen to screen. He additionally included a few quizzes that functioned by requiring the learner to move text on the screen from one location to another to match with the correct answers. How do you think this eLearning module was received by the learning audience? Do you think that people can only learn if training is presented using their learning style?

Introduction

Learning theory might seem a bit intimidating, but learning theories are simply the published end-result of observations and research on how people best learn. Each researcher approaches learning in a slightly different way, resulting in many unique theories about how people intake and process information. In reality, many learning professionals have a favorite learning theory that they use frequently, but there is no single learning theory that will provide optimal learning outcomes in every learning situation. Therefore, it is important to understand each of the most commonly used learning theories because the selected learning theory will influence and guide how training is designed, developed, and evaluated [1]. Some of the earliest learning theories were developed before we had multiple ways to view and evaluate learning [2]. With the advent of modern technology, the science of brain-based learning provides new insight into how people learn, and modern technology can help researchers actually view the brain during the learning process [3].

In addition to guiding the design and development of training, learning theories can also serve to frame the evaluation of training. For example, if training is based on

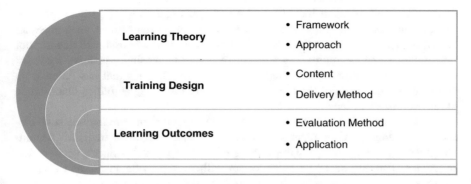

Learning Theory	• Framework • Approach
Training Design	• Content • Delivery Method
Learning Outcomes	• Evaluation Method • Application

Fig. 5.1 Relationship of learning theory to design and outcomes

a particular learning theory, training that uses that theoretical approach should produce a certain the expected response from the learner (Fig. 5.1). The expected response forms the basis for evaluation of the training design, and the skill of the designer and instructor will be used a certain way when a particular learning theory guides training. There are many books and resources that go into great detail about each of the learning theories, but the purpose of this chapter is to provide a general overview of the most commonly used learning theories used for training design and development.

Learning Theories and Frameworks

Behaviorism

Behaviorism is one of the older learning theories, developed over the late 19th and early twentieth century. At that time, the ultimate output of learning was a change in performance, therefore behaviorism focused on changing the behavior of the learner [4]. Many are familiar with the story of Pavlov and his experimental approach that caused dogs to salivate each time they heard a bell ring. This conditioned response occurred because initially the dogs were given meat powder at the same time that they heard a bell ring. Over time, just the sound of the bell triggered the salivatory response even when there was no meat powder reward. From this early experimental research came the concept of classical conditioning, which is defined as a direct transfer of the response towards one stimulus, the meat powder, to that of another stimulus, the sound of a bell.

Building on the early work of Pavlov, the concept of operant conditioning expanded on classical conditioning by introducing positive and negative rewards to reinforce performance of the desired behavior. From an educational perspective, the instruction determines the desired behavior of the learner and institutes positive or negative rewards to reinforce the behavior. Positive reinforcement is the introduction of something positive to reinforce repetition of the desired behavior. Examples of positive reinforcement include grades and skills exercises. Negative reinforcement is not providing punishment, but rather involves removal of an unpleasant stimulus such as canceling the additional homework that was assigned due to poor performance, seeing improved grades, or receiving increasingly positive feedback about behavior. Although behaviorism is one of the theories that has fallen from frequent use, elements of the theory can be seen in learning activities that include skills exercises and repetitive drills.

Health information training that is based on behaviorism may include such elements as graded quizzes, repetition of skills exercises, prizes or treats for demonstrating desired behaviors, and the training will include clear learning objectives and outcomes. Training based on behaviorism will often provide strong and frequent encouragement and praise when movement in the right direction is observed, or when goals are achieved to further motivate the learner. One of the pitfalls of behaviorism is that when praise is not provided for accomplished goals, the learner may not experience reinforcement of the desired behavior, which can negate learning [5].

Cognitivism

While behaviorism focused on changed behavior as evidence of learning, many questions about how people learn were left unanswered. Cognitivism emerged in the mid-twentieth century as a way to explain the process of how people learn. The theory of cognitivism proposed that learning not only changes behavior but involves how information is organized in the brain [4]. Cognitivism focuses on the mechanics of memory, proposing that information is encoded in the brain when stimulus in the environment reaches the attention of the brain. From there, the large amount of encoded information taken into the brain is filtered so that irrelevant information is removed, and then the newly encoded information is stored in short term memory. New information stored in short-term memory will only remain for 20-30 seconds unless transferred to long term memory. Additionally, information can only be integrated into short term memory in small pieces, which is why telephone numbers and social security numbers were developed to be only seven to ten digits long.

An easy way to visualize cognitivism is to picture the brain as a large filing cabinet. In this mental filing cabinet, new information must be coded and filed with like information so that it is placed into context and can be retrieved at a later time. To move new information into long-term memory, the information in short-term memory is encoded a second time to group it with like information so that it can be retrieved at a later time, based on each person's unique mental labels and internal brain filing systems. Using a foundation of cognitive learning, in 1965 Gagne proposed nine events of instruction that must be present for new knowledge to be encoded and moved into long-term memory [6]. The nine events of instruction include (1) gaining the attention of the learner through a stimulus, (2) providing the objective of the learning, (3) connecting new knowledge with previously acquired knowledge, (4) presenting material in a way that is clear and memorable, (5) directing learning that is to occur, (6) allowing for performance of the new knowledge, (7) presenting feedback on the learning process, (8) assessing use of the new knowledge with additional feedback, and (9) allowing for practice to promote the ability for future retrieval of the new knowledge. The steps within Gagne's nine events of learning allow for encoding and retrieval of new knowledge.

Health information training that is designed using cognitive learning theory might include techniques that help the learners remember new information by creating strong connections with existing knowledge. Training techniques may include repetition of concepts, using mnemonics, imagery, and unusual associations that help the learner to recall information because it is tied to something unusual or unexpected.

Social Cognitivism

Around the same time that behaviorism was emerging, theorists were starting to examine how learning occurred within a cultural and social context. Researchers noted that learners were influenced by their language and culture when learning, and that the interplay of teachers and peers helped learners to test new ideas. The goal of social cognitivism is to help the learner grow from dependence to independence when learning new information by using the influence of the teacher and peers to support the learning and growth process [7].

Health information technology training that is developed using the foundation of social cognitive theory may include the opportunity for students to identify their goals for learning. And included in the training should be time for peer interaction and discussion about what has been learned, and opportunities to practice new skills that help to establish and maintain independence.

Social Learning Theory

Social learning theory emerged in the early twentieth century and was developed in recognition of the importance of the environment on learning. The ability to observe, imitate, and learn a new behavior contributes to the learning process. For social learning to occur, the student must be able to observe or pay attention, process and retain what is learned in memory, and possess the motivation to observe and imitate another's behavior [8].

When social learning is the foundation of health information technology training, the class may be structured as a flipped classroom where the learners are given prework. The prework includes information that is later discussed with peers in the classroom. Training using the social learning model will have minimal instructor activity and a large amount of learner interactivity. Social learning can also occur when a learner imitates the behavior and processes of a preceptor in the real-world environment.

Humanism

The learning theory of humanism emerged at the same time that psychology was developing theories about self-esteem and human potential, including Maslow's hierarchy of needs theory. Training that is designed using humanism presupposes that learning is a personal decision made to help one achieve their full potential. Humanism uses five principles to guide education that include (1) self-direction and independence, (2) assuming responsibility for what is learned, (3) growth of creativity, (4) curiosity, and (5) inclusion of the arts. Humanism forms some of the core elements of adult learning theory, which will be presented later in this chapter [1].

When humanism is the foundation for health information technology training, there will be an emphasis on the benefits of obtaining training including professional growth and the relationship between training and optimal patient care. Additionally, training using humanism as an approach may offer options for the learner to select when their training occurs as well as the methods for obtaining training. Emphasis will also be placed on linking the outcomes of learning to the benefits of new knowledge and professional responsibility.

Constructivism

The theory of constructivism proposes that learning occurs not when information is provided to the learner, but when the learner reflects on the new information and tests that new information by interacting with others. The knowledge gained is shaped by the learner's own past experiences and attitudes, and the input of peers helps to validate or test new learning. As constructivism gained acceptance, later theorists proposed an experiential learning model that progresses from concrete experiences to reflection on the experience, development of additional concepts based on the reflection, and finally testing of the new concepts developed in the learner's environment [5]. Constructivism is primarily used as underpinning for adult learning because the learner must have a certain level of experience and context to process and reflect on new information.

When the learning theory of constructivism is used for health information technology training, the learning event may include activities that promote reflection on new information such as questions and answers about new information, practice time in the classroom, opportunities for independent practice in a safe *sandbox* environment, and the ability to interact with experienced users of the new technology.

Brain-Based Learning

Scientists and researchers are now able to view how the brain functions during the learning process. Hart initially proposed the theory of brain-based learning in 1983 [3]. The theory of brain-based learning proposes that the brain changes as learning occurs by forming new neurons and synapses between neurons. Interestingly, the newly formed connections and neurons help the learner to organize new information within the neural networks. Another term used for the growth and changes seen in the brain during learning is neuroplasticity. Through technology, researchers have seen that learning engages certain areas of the brain, and not all areas of the brain are engaged in learning. When learning is occurring, the brain produces adrenaline and serotonin to facilitate the work and growth of neurons. In addition to facilitating learning, these neurotransmitters may also produce a change in mood or emotion as learning occurs.

The brain learns best when certain elements are incorporated into the training such as practice and engagement with the emotions of the learner. However, negative emotions such as fear of failure or punishment and social humiliation can inhibit learning and create a fight or flight response to training. Learning occurs when emotions are carefully balanced to provide a learning challenge without excess frustration [3]. Instructors should be alert for learners that appear overwhelmed during the learning event and intervene with a later or different training opportunity if needed.

Training that is based on brain-based learning may include pre-training communication and information that helps to inform, excite and reduce stress for learners. Classrooms will be engaging but non-judgmental, with plenty of positive feedback. Instructors may monitor learner stress levels and provide breaks and methods for reducing stress such as games or social interaction opportunities.

Adult Learning Theory

Although referred to as a theory, adult learning theory is more of a framework that arose from an exploration of many learning theories applied specifically to adult learners. In contrast to the adult learning framework, the science of teaching children is called pedagogy. Pedagogy is primarily focused on providing foundational new information and knowledge to children, usually through a unidirectional flow of information from teacher to learner. Andragogy, or adult learning, is based on the idea that adults have a lifetime of learning and experience and must be participants in their own learning [9]. Andragogy is based on six premises, and Table 5.1 provides a comparison of pedagogy versus andragogy.

While andragogy does not explain how people learn, it does provide insight into creating the conditions that allow adults to best learn. Although it is tempting to utilize andragogy for all adult learning, there are appropriate times and situations where a pedagogical approach or a mixed approach may be the best model for delivering training, especially when presenting new information that is not yet aligned with a life or work context.

Health information technology training that is based on andragogy may include the following elements. The need for training and the purpose of training is clearly communicated early and often. During the training event, learners are presented

Table 5.1 Pedagogy versus andragogy

Pedagogy	Andragogy
The learner needs knowledge, but only what is needed to reach a defined competency such as to pass a test	The learner wants to know why learning is necessary before investing the time and energy into pursuing learning
The teacher views the learner as a dependent learner, and the teacher must provide the information that is to be learned	Adults have life experiences and are accustomed to being responsible for their own decisions. Adults tend to resist learning that they perceive is forced upon them.
The instruction does not relate to, nor consider the learner's past experiences. The final authority is the textbook or other authoritative source of information.	Adults have a great volume of life experience and appreciate learning experiences that acknowledge the value of their past experiences.
The learner will learn only that which the teacher tells them they must learn in order to achieve a goal or competency.	Adults seek to learn those things that will prepare them for situations or tasks that are imminent; and seek learning that will help them progress in life or accomplish tasks more readily.
Learning is ordered and grouped by subject and therefore has little relation to the logic of life experiences	Adults learn best when information is presented or aligned with the context of life or life situations
Learners are motivated to learn by extrinsic forces such as teacher approval or grades	The greatest motivator for adult learning is intrinsic rather than extrinsic.

with information about why the training is important and how it aligns with organizational strategy and enhances personal development and growth. Instructors may take the time to relate new concepts such as documenting vital signs in the EHR to prior experiences of documenting vital signs within a paper chart. Learners may also be given the choice of when to attend a learning event and possibly to select different learning delivery methods such as eLearning versus a classroom learning session.

Learning Styles

In the early 1990s the concept of learning styles overtook the education and training world. The premise of learning styles what that people learn best when they receive instruction through their own learning style [10]. The four learning styles of visual, aural, read/write, and kinesthetic were embedded into classrooms, and training experts were sometimes tasked with developing four different training programs to meet the needs of each type of learner. However, ongoing research has shown that student learning is not impacted either way when learning is presented using their learning style versus another learning style.

The latest research indicates that people may have a preferred way of learning, so that if they like words more than images, or hearing better than reading, learning outcomes are not influenced by how the learning is presented but the learner may prefer a certain method of presentation. Although incorporating different learning approaches to meet every learning style is not necessary for improved learning, using variation in training delivery methods may help to stimulate and maintain engagement with a learning event. Although it has been demonstrated that learners can learn through methods other than their favorite or preferred learning style, training that is designed to engage learners through many different methods such as listening, viewing, reading, and doing aligns with the need for the brain to frequently shift focus, and will engage each learner more deeply when their learning preference is presented. To incorporate learning preferences into training, learning professionals can provide a break for the human brain about every twenty minutes by seamlessly switching the delivery method, a technique that may help learners remain engaged.

The Science of Instruction

Research has been conducted on the science of instruction for eLearning, which is often the delivery method for health information technology training. Researchers have focused on best practices for training design when eLearning is the delivery method. Some of the principles developed by Clark R and Mayer R [11] directly impact how eLearning should be designed through the use of evidence and best practices.

Some of the key findings from this research include the greater learning impact of using words and images rather than words alone, and making sure that the words are placed close to the visual graphics to minimize eye movement can also facilitate better learning. Another import discovery for eLearning developers is that information is received through either the eyes or the ears, but the brain cannot use both pathways at the same time. Looking back at John's training design at the beginning of this chapter, this means that John was actually creating cognitive overload and brain fatigue by narrating word for word the same words shown on the screen. By adding arrows that needed to be clicked to move forward in the eLearning, John also included extraneous actions that detract from learning. Any extraneous images included in the eLearning created by John will also detract from learning. Images must be relevant and associated with the content.

E-learning for HIT training that is based on the science of instruction should avoid the use of extraneous motion or images that do not relate to the content. Fatiguing eye motion should be reduced by placing explanatory text near images, and screens should contain either text or narration, but avoid word for word narration of the text. Screens should be designed to avoid clutter and also include plenty of white space to reduce brain fatigue. The focus of the science of instruction is to minimize brain fatigue and cognitive overload by reducing unnecessary eye movements and decreasing the need for the brain to process irrelevant information.

Summary

Learning theories were developed to help explain how to change behavior and to explain how people learn, thus providing the ability to create the conditions that facilitate optimal learning. While no single learning theory perfectly addresses the process of learning, each theory contains elements that can be used to support successful training design and effective learning. In addition, the use of a particular learning theory can guide the approach to learning evaluation and management.

The process of training can be highly impactful to both an organization and to a learner. When training is not designed using the evidence that can produce the best outcomes, the time spent in learning may create negative outcomes or waste organizational resources. In today's environment, health care workers have many options for their employment and careers. Effective training can not only support and develop a successful professional career, but can create a positive attitude towards change and the use of health information technology in the provision of health care.

Discussion Questions and Answers

1. Using the cognitive learning theory, list some ways to help learners encode information to move it into short term memory.

   (a) Use mnemonics to help learners associate a concept with another word
   (b) Use images to encode new concepts for short-term memory
   (c) Make sure that information is not too long to be retained in short-term memory
   (d) Relate new information to existing knowledge
   (e) Use repetition

2. Which learning theory(s) fit best with HIT training and why?

   (a) Learners can select their own preferences here

3. What types of activities would you include in a class that is based on social cognitivism?

   (a) Have students identify learning goals
   (b) Allow time for peer interaction and discussion
   (c) Provide time for learners to practice new skills

4. How would you structure the design of content when using the adult learning framework?

   (a) Allow for learners to select their preferred class time for learning
   (b) Communicate the reason for training
   (c) Relate new concepts to existing experience
   (d) Provide learners the choice of learning delivery method

5. What are three differences between pedagogy and andragogy?

Pedagogy	Andragogy
The learner needs knowledge, but only what is needed to reach a defined competency such as to pass a test	The learner wants to know why learning is necessary before investing the time and energy into pursuing learning
The teacher views the learner as a dependent learner, and the teacher must provide the information that is to be learned.	Adults have life experiences and are accustomed to being responsible for their own decisions. Adults tend to resist learning that they perceive is forced upon them.
The instruction does not relate to, nor consider the learner's past experiences. The final authority is the textbook or other authoritative source of information.	Adults have a great volume of life experience and appreciate learning experiences that acknowledge the value of their past experiences.
The learner will learn only that which the teacher tells them they must learn in order to achieve a goal or competency.	Adults seek to learn those things that will prepare them for situations or tasks that are imminent; and seek learning that will help them progress in life or accomplish tasks more readily.
Learning is ordered and grouped by subject and therefore has little relation to the logic of life experiences	Adults learn best when information is presented or aligned with the context of life or life situations
Learners are motivated to learn by extrinsic forces such as teacher approval or grades	The greatest motivator for adult learning is intrinsic rather than extrinsic.

References

1. Wu WH, Chiou WB, Kao HY, Hu CHA, Huang SH. Re-exploring game-assisted learning research: the perspective of learning theoretical bases. Comput Educ. 2012;59(4):1153–61. https://doi.org/10.1016/j.compedu.2012.05.003.
2. Ertmer PA, Newby TJ. Behaviorism, cognitivism, constructivism: comparing critical features from an instructional design perspective. Perform Improv Q. 2013;26(2):43–71. https://doi.org/10.1002/piq.21143.
3. Thompson S (2019) Brain-based learning. *Brain-Based Learning—Research Starters Education*, 1-1.
4. Clark KR. Learning theories: cognitivism. Radiol Technol. 2018;90(2):176–9.
5. Younas A. Learning curve. Strengthening creativity in nurse educators. Nursing. 2018;48(5):15–6.
6. Ullah H, Rehman AU, Bibi S. Gagné's 9 events of instruction—a time tested way to improve teaching. Pak Armed Forces Med J. 2015;65(4):535–9.
7. Austin RT. Organisational theories of human learning and employee development initiatives. J Social Psychol Sci. 2015;8(1):8–15.
8. Brieger E, Arghode V, McLean G. Connecting theory and practice: reviewing six learning theories to inform online instruction. Eur J Train Dev. 2020;44(4/5):321–39. https://doi.org/10.1108/EJTD-07-2019-0116.
9. Knowles MS, Holton EF III, Swanson RA. The adult learner: the definitive classic in adult education and human resources development. Elsevier Butterworth Heinemann; 2005.
10. Anderson J. A conceptual framework of a study in preferred learning styles: pedagogy or andragogy. Spalding University; 2007.

11. Clark R, Mayer R. e-Learning and the science of instruction: proven guidelines for consumers and designers of multimedia learning, 4th ed. Wiley; 2016. ISBN: 978-1-119-15866-0. March 2016. p. 528.

Brenda Kulhanek is an associate professor at the Vanderbilt University School of Nursing and has a history of leadership in both informatics and clinical education. Dr. Kulhanek holds a PhD from Capella University and a doctor of nursing practice (DNP) from Walden University. She is board certified in nursing informatics, nursing professional development, and executive leadership. Her publications include informatics textbook chapters and multiple informatics articles. She recently participated in the Scope & Standards for Nursing Informatics publication. She teaches informatics at the master's and doctoral levels and has a particular interest in strengthening nursing through nursing informatics education, and the integration of informatics into practice to support improvement of patient outcomes.

Chapter 6
Generational Differences in Training

Kathleen Mandato

Abstract Understanding generational differences in learning can help positively impact training. Each generation has a preferred method of learning that should be considered when developing training, and there are some common approaches that can be used that can enhance training for all generations. This chapter will provide insight and best practices for training multiple generations of learners.

Keywords Generations · Mature · Baby boomer · Generation X · Millennial Generation Y · Generation Z · Microlearning · Learning preferences · Digital mind Cognitive overload · Multi-tasking · Technology-based instruction · Intergenerational learning

Learning Outcomes
1. Discuss the impact of generational differences on training approaches
2. Identify learning needs based on generational differences
3. Explain training approaches based on generational differences

K. Mandato (✉)
Epic Training and Delivery and Administrative/Nursing Fellowship Program, Vanderbilt University Medical Center, Nashville, TN, USA

B. Kulhanek, K. Mandato (eds.), *Healthcare Technology Training*, Health Informatics, https://doi.org/10.1007/978-3-031-10322-3_6

A Generational Difference

Several years ago, I was teaching an undergraduate class focused on adults returning to continue their studies. The class consisted of various generations, some were just beginning their careers, and others had worked in health care for many years. I was teaching a class on Electronic Health Records (EHR). During the class, I introduced a learning tool that was provided by the textbook publisher which presented additional learning activities, practice exercises and EHR simulations. I provided a step-by-step set of directions for how to access the web site as well as a special code that was needed to register on the web site for these additional learning activities. Soon I began to receive multiple emails and text messages from students who were not able to access the site, did not have a code that worked, and many other issues. I reiterated in a communication to the class the need to read the steps I had provided very carefully and use the proper codes where needed. Each student had received a code of their own with their textbooks, so some students were using the enrollment code in place of the student code, and vice versa.

During this situation, my observations were that most of the younger generation of students were comfortable following the steps to access the additional learning activities. Many of the older generation were struggling and requested that someone walk them through the steps to access the web site. As a result, I dedicated the last 30 minutes of class to help those that were struggling. The group of older students walked down the hall to an available computer lab, and I had them all follow the steps together, one by one. Aside from one person truly having an invalid code, the class did well and overall felt more comfortable now that they knew how to log in and access the activities.

The important lesson learned through this experience was that not everyone is comfortable with technology. When introducing technology, it is important to provide very clear guidance and directions. In this case, a micro learning lesson that demonstrated the step-by-step process for accessing the learning system would have been very helpful, especially for visual learners. In a situation where a live person is not available, as was the case when I began to teach this same class online a few months later, having a micro learning lesson and a clear set of directions helped to ease the learners' concerns. In addition, I learned that it is important for students to have resources available to help themselves. As a result, I now provide the technology assistance support line in my directions, so they can have a person walk them through the process. Lastly, I learned that it is extremely important to explain upfront the purpose of why the learners need to follow a certain process, in this case to access an ancillary system. For this ancillary activity, the learners were required to complete a few tutorials and then complete a simulation which required them to work through common EHR documentation scenarios. Being able to understand the direct connection between the extra activities and what they represented helped the students to grasp the importance of the assignments and the need for technology to access them.

Introduction

When we examine the learning audiences of today, one of the first things that comes to mind are the various generations that exist in the workplace. Currently, the oldest employees in the workplace are separated from the youngest people in the workplace by over 55 years. Research shows that each generation has their own unique learning preferences and failure to incorporate generational differences into training design can result in learning with decreased effectiveness and frustrated learners [1]. The purpose of this chapter is to explore generational differences and how they impact learning approaches for health information technology training that fits all learners.

The 5 Generations

Generations are based not only on age, but on shared experiences for those within each age category [1]. In the workforce of today, there are five generations that make up different age groups of learners (Table 6.1). According to the World Press, a generation is defined as, "a group of individuals born around the same time who share specific attitudes and values that can influence their behavior and expectations at work" ([2] p. 3).

Table 6.1 Generational characteristics and learning preferences

Generation	Characteristics & learning preference
Matures/ traditionalists 1925–1945	• Appreciate face-to-face interaction • Gravitates toward consistency, logic and discipline • Likes to be recognized for qualifications and experience • Likes to learn by watching and then doing
Baby boomers 1946–1966	• Values hard work • Sees training as a benefit to help them in their careers • Can do either face-to face or online training-prefers face-to face
Generation X 1965–1985	• They value their autonomy • Prefer online, self-paced learning that allows them to learn by doing • They like to provide feedback and suggestions on content of training/ have a say
Generation Y 1981–2000	• Hard working and achievement oriented • Enjoys fast-moving and interactive activities as well as social media • They like to collaborate with peers • Prefers to use technology to learn
Generation Z 1995–2010	• Most adept at handling technology • Prefers to learn by see and do • Like recorded lectures and viewing online study guides • Watches videos all the time • Prefers interactive learning in person or online

Matures

The Matures, also known as the Traditionalists, were born between 1925 and 1945. This generation lived through the Great Depression and felt the effects of World War II. Their experience with technology may be limited to what was around during that period such as radio signals and phonographs [3]. While this generation demonstrates flexibility and the willingness to adapt in order to support an organization, they seem to appreciate face to face interaction versus learning with technology [4]. This group also appreciates consistency, logic and discipline [2].

Baby Boomers

The Baby Boomers were born between 1946 and 1966 and currently represent around 44% of the workforce [5]. This generation experienced many cultural changes associated with the Vietnam War and the subsequent economic boom. During this time, women started entering the workforce and the civil rights movement was emerging. The Baby Boomer generation values hard work and views training as a benefit. They look for how training will enhance their work skills and make them more productive. Baby Boomers are open to technology but prefer face to face interaction and view technology as a means to an end [2].

Generation X

Members of Generation X were born between 1965 and 1985. This generation is known as the "latch key kids" and has lived through a recession, economic instability, and corporate downsizing. This generation saw the development of computers and lived through the AIDS epidemic [2]. They are fiercely independent and value their autonomy. The preferred learning style for Generation X is to learn by doing. This generation will gravitate toward computer self-paced learning versus instructor-led sessions. They also like to have a say in the content of the training.

Generation Y

Those in Generation Y, or Millennials as they are often termed, were born between 1980 and 2000. This generation is hard working and achievement oriented. Millennials are digital natives and accustomed to maneuvering through technology quickly while multitasking. They are largely committed to institutional learning and value moral and ethical principles. Millennials enjoy fast-moving and interactive activities as well as social media. Millennials prefer a more collaborative learning environment where they can interact with their peers, and this generation likes the use of technology for learning and often rely on their phones as resources [2].

Generation Z

The youngest generation in the workplace is Generation Z, born between 2000 and 2010. This generation was born into technology, and they view technology as a normal part of life. They are the most adept at handling technology as they have never known any other way. Members of Generation Z thrive in a collaborative environment, and they enjoy learning by seeing and doing. This generation likes recorded lectures and viewing online study guides. Those in Generation Z spend a great amount of time watching videos and they prefer learning that is interactive whether in person or online [2].

Trends Identified across Generations

Digital Mind

Understanding the characteristics of the five generations will help in offering a blend of options that will create the ideal learning environment. All generations have become reliant to a certain degree on digital technology. Examples of reliance on digital technology include seeking input from multiple sources, and the expectation that information can be quickly obtained. Digital media and devices have transformed the way people live and learn and as a result, learners may think and process information differently. The term *digital mind* refers to how people process information and learn new information. It will be critical to develop classroom activities that can accommodate learning styles associated with digital minds [6].

Strategies for Teaching

One of the key elements for effective learning for all generations is engaging the learner. The learner must make a commitment to move forward and learn the content being offered. Being aware of generational differences can help reflect different thinking and attitudes and life experiences about technology. Instructors can use this information to provide different options for learning that do not involve technology, although technology-enhanced learning is ubiquitous in the training industry.

The first generational teaching strategy, according to Brown [7] and Driscoll [8] is to focus on outcomes rather than techniques. This strategy involves facilitating students to work through information in such a way that the learner is solving a problem and learning at the same time. Also known as reality-based learning, this concept centers around having students work through realistic scenarios that will help them perform their job. The benefit of this type of learning is that the learner can actively use their digital minds to uncover knowledge and then apply it to a scenario through active learning.

Reality-based training can be employed in most healthcare settings during initial training sessions that are focused on learning to use the electronic medical record. Once the foundational training is initiated, the learner can use a training patient and provider to review key steps needed for documenting in the electronic medical record. A *playground* or test environment can allow the learner to work through different scenarios such as documenting a patient's vitals, completing a history and physical, or documenting a visit note without impacting live patient data. A practice workbook outlining scenarios and workflows and access to a playground environment can allow for learners to practice independently outside of the classroom. This technique helps reinforce what was learned during the training as well as to build muscle memory.

Another strategy for multi-generational training according to Brown [7] and Driscoll [8] is to offer more than one option for delivering content. This can be as simple as providing an electronic workbook for learners to follow along while the instructor is facilitating the technology related content using either a virtual or an in-person classroom setting. An additional technique to consider is to have the instructor walk through the workflow in the playground environment while the learners are also following along in their own playground environment. This method is successful either in a virtual or in-person setting and allows the learners to see the workflow and processes modeled so that they can imitate the same behaviors and processes. The flipped classroom approach can also provide another option for blended learning. In the flipped classroom approach, learners are introduced to new content prior to meeting in a classroom. Armed with this pre-class preparation, learners can utilize classroom time to discuss and practice the content with their peers in a classroom setting. The flipped classroom format of learning delivery offers two different methods for learning and practicing content, through self-learning and through group discussion and practice.

Multi-Tasking

Learners from the Millennial Generation and Generation Y are proficient at multi-tasking and are accustomed to doing more than one thing at the same time. These generations have always had the internet and cell phone available and are highly adept at using technology. These learners can deal with many streams of information coming in at once and prefer learning through multitasking. It is important for instructors to acknowledge the learning preferences of these generations and offer opportunities for learners to multitask. An example of multitasking incorporated into the classroom would be to have students answer questions while listening to an online podcast or take notes while watching a video [7, 8].

Visual Format/Emphasizing Key Points

Based on the technology and internet capabilities of today, younger generations of learners prefer to utilize technology to find information and to learn about new concepts on the internet. These learners look for visual cues commonly found on the internet such as headers, side headers and highlighted text. Formatting plays a big part in how information is processed, and decisions are made, and they depend on these formatting elements to quickly navigate to the desired information. As an instructor, consider helping these learners to recognize important information rather than depend on headlines and visual cues by emphasizing the need to slow down and take the time to recognize and absorb the details of what is important [7, 8].

Interactive Groups

A trend prevalent across generations is the collaborative mindset. Many learners prefer group activities and value the interaction gained from such experiences. Working in groups is important because it helps to encourage engagement as well as promote diverse and different ideas within a group. Diverse input can spark new ideas and promote learning. Additionally, relationships can form within interactive groups that will help learners establish future contacts for ongoing discussion outside of the classroom. Learners frequently seek out other learners that have been in their learning groups to ask them questions later. Despite a preference for collaborative learning and recognition of the value of learning from peers, be aware that in some cases, learners may gravitate toward peer opinions over that of their instructors. Instructors should seek to validate the final consensus emanating from group learning to ensure that course learning outcomes remain accurate and correct [9].

Reflection

Because digital minds are used to working in a fast-paced environment, they need to take some time to stop and reflect on what they have learned. Promoting a time for reflection can help learners take this pause in their busy schedules to process the information they have learned. According to Burton, p. 2 (2016), "reflection helps us connect the act of doing with the act of learning." For the process of reflection to be fully successful, it is recommended that opportunities for reflection occur prior to training, during training, and after the learning experience [10].

Technology Based Instruction

Technology based instruction can be described as learning that is delivered using technology. This can include a wide variety of methods, such as computer-based training, simulations, e-learning, virtual reality training, gamification, and podcasts. Research suggests that the younger generations are more likely to be comfortable with technology, while older generations may need more encouragement to participate in this type of learning [2].

When training learners to use the electronic medical record, which is technology, technology is used to train technology. The goal of technology-based training is that learners will be able to apply the new knowledge and skills gained from on-the-job training. The primary goal of technology training is for learners to not only demonstrate the ability to use the technology that they will use to perform their job duties, but also for learners to understand how to find critical resources that can help them with functionality if needed. Due to the recent COVID pandemic, many classrooms have shifted from an in-person model to a remote learning approach using communication applications such as Zoom, Skype or Teams to deliver training. This shift to remote technology has created a new opportunity to develop new content that is more dynamic and interactive. Multigenerational learners are gravitating toward this type of learning because they not only can listen and follow along with the instructor but also engage online with the content, and work on practice exercises and complete quizzes.

The reason that a high-tech approach to learning appeals to multiple generations of learners is that the training and classroom settings are more interactive and provide opportunities for increased interaction. Learners often have the flexibility to communicate with the instructor during or after class via chat, email, or text messaging. An additional benefit of a high tech, distance learning model that appeals to all generations is that the learner becomes more accountable for their learning. Finally, the learners can employ technology in the privacy of their own home and learn in a comfortable and familiar home environment.

Blended Approaches

Some learners, especially those from earlier generations, may prefer to be face-to-face with an instructor in a physical classroom setting. Technology can help make this happen without requiring the learner or instructor to be physically present in the same space. With communication technologies such as Zoom or Skype, learners can see and interact with the instructor in real time while online. Instructors that are physically in a classroom can also use these same communication technologies to record a learning session while teaching to students that are attending remotely. By having a camera in the classroom, remote students can watch instructors facilitating, answering questions within the classroom, and presenting key topics.

Depending on the organization and environmental considerations, learners may also be able to attend class in person and then finish the rest of the learning or practice exercises at home. For those working in an environment where technology is embedded into daily work, a culture of continual learning and growth is imperative. To cultivate a culture of learning and continuous growth, some key practices should be considered. In the following examples, learning is illustrated in a way that appeals to multi-generational learners and should be utilized as standard operating procedures in order to establish a rich learning environment across multiple generations [2].

Continuous Learning

Many successful organizations attribute some of their success to learning programs that have been put in place to support continuous education. Continuous education or learning can be delivered in different formats. Examples of successful formats that incorporate continuous learning into a workplace culture include having employees taking a time out to watch a quick video on patient safety, accessing a short job aide, or reading an article on the latest technology employed in the organization. Based on these examples, it is important to provide an online repository for job aides, articles, and quick guides that are available to learners at any time to help them navigate through the EHR as well as other organizational systems and processes. The multi-generational appeal of this just-in-time material is that it is quick and easy to retrieve from an always-available online resource [11].

As with any learning, care needs to be taken to ensure that the brain is not overloaded with too much content during training. Based on the Cognitive Load Theory (CLT), humans have limited working memory capacity and can only absorb a certain amount of information in each learning session [2]. Technology based instruction can pose a challenge in this regard due to the amount of information presented and the ease or difficulty with navigating the system. The presence of a readily available repository of learning materials allows learners to fill in the gaps of their knowledge with additional information and instruction when they are ready and able to learn more.

Personalization of Learning

Research has shown that each learner has a personalized learning preferences and style that is based on how they best receive information and knowledge and on what has worked best for them in past learning [11]. Offering multiple options or a menu of choices for learning new content, skills or tools will allow for a more personalized approach to learning [11]. Examples of this include offering online or in-person learning opportunities and interactive eLearning modules. All these training formats allow for the learner to master new content in a way that works best for them. Creating a menu of multiple approaches to training delivery does require more work and resources on the part of the training team and different training options may be restricted if resources are limited. Individualized learning that contains real-life scenarios helps adult learners to make a connection with the materials being presented and allows for immediate application of theory into practice [12].

Intergenerational Learning

Organizations are looking for approaches and strategies that help to integrate multiple generations into the workplace. One type of strategy that can help with this is reverse mentoring. Reverse mentoring is an established practice where a younger junior employee is put in a role to mentor and share expertise with an older senior colleague. Mentorship is based on intergenerational learning and allows knowledge to be passed on from one generation to another [2]. However, in this situation, the roles are reversed and instead of a senior colleague mentoring a junior colleague, the opposite occurs so that the junior colleague can share technical or topic expertise, especially on technology related topics. Reverse mentoring was introduced by Jack Welch, former CEO of General Electric, in 1999 [2] and has become a best practice in many large organizations to encourage knowledge sharing. Reverse mentoring additionally encourages organizations to capitalize on generational differences and similarities by recognizing the strengths of each generation and building upon them.

Microlearning

Microlearning can be described as short bursts of content delivered to learners through a variety of delivery methods that include text, images, videos, audio, tests, quizzes and games [13]. One of the reasons why microlearning is becoming popular has to do with the sheer volume of information that is available. Because information is readily accessible and easily retrievable, the attention spans of learners are decreasing [14]. Keeping shorter attention spans in mind means that training needs to be about more than just gaining the knowledge that is already available to learners through technology. Training needs to be about engaging the learner and helping the learner to apply their new knowledge at any time and in any situation. Microlearning helps provide succinct learning that is preferred by multigenerational learners who want to be in control of their learning pathways.

Age-Diverse Audiences

There are many best practices that outline how to successfully accommodate a multigenerational class of learners. These same learning needs and preferences for age diverse audiences must be considered when designing or facilitating technology-based training. Following are some basic tips and suggestions for ensuring that all ages, especially the learning needs of older adults, are accommodated from a learning perspective.

The first step in designing effective multi-generational training is to make sure that a proper needs assessment has been conducted prior to developing the training. During this stage, an in-depth analysis of the learning audience is conducted, additional details on the analysis process can be found in Chap. 8. As a result of the needs assessment, the demographics of the learning audience are determined, and age-inclusive factors can guide how training content is delivered. It is important to ensure that screens are large enough to accommodate vision needs, and that seating is comfortable for all learners for long periods of time. Any known disabilities should be accommodated using technology such as screen readers or speech recognition applications. Because learning engages all senses, environmental factors play a big role in the successful delivery of training.

An additional best practice for learners that may be technologically challenged is to offer a basic computer navigation class. However, time and resources may present a barrier for providing this type of preparation for health information technology training. To help with resource challenges, basic computer navigation classes can be delivered through an in-person experience or through an online learning module. For those learners who have had little experience using technology, a basic computer navigation course can be very beneficial. A basic computer navigation course typically includes basic processes such as how to open and close a computer window, how to use a mouse, and a few introductory steps of how to log on to the communication technology that will be utilized for ongoing courses.

Despite the additional time and resources needed for providing a basic computer navigation course, the new knowledge gained can help ease the minds of the learners and reduce anxiety, set the learners up for success, and help them know what they can expect so that there are no surprises. When the learner is a little more comfortable with the technology being offered, they will demonstrate additional commitment and confidence to practice what has been learned. A microlearning lesson may be a perfect option to help learners understand what to expect when they proceed to the main training course. Micro-learning can also be used to demonstrate how to log into the communication technology for class using a step-by-step demonstration of the process.

It is important to maintain structure in the delivery of training, especially when dealing with age-diverse audiences. Providing clear learning objectives and an explanation of how the training will be delivered upfront can help ease any anxiety that may be present on the part of the learner. In addition, as with any adult learner, providing resources will help the learner understand where to go if questions come up. Emphasizing critical information as well as providing reminders on key points can help promote important concepts for retention. Finally, presenting information in segments or chunks allows learners to process information and experience a more meaningful learning event.

Learners of all generations respond positively to feedback as it builds confidence and helps learners understand how they are progressing with mastering the main concepts and learning objectives in training. Mentors or subject matter experts (SMEs) can enhance training by helping learners understand the relevance of the knowledge they are gaining related to what their job tasks will be. In addition, having someone available to help monitor the learner's practice during a training session will help validate that the learner is grasping the necessary concepts. Although older generations are more used to the *sage on the stage* approach to learning, the younger generation of learners prefer the *guide on the side* approach to training.

Conclusion

Awareness of generational perspectives and increased understanding of those differences can help build a more robust learning experience. Improved learning experiences ultimately lead to a more productive organization that benefits from enhanced understanding among the generations. The goal of multi-generational training is to encourage commitment from each generation of learners from the instructor's perspectives to focusing on what is important to the learner. Generational awareness can help instructors achieve that goal by being aware of the traits associated with each generation. With generational awareness, instructors can utilize different techniques to enhance the learning environment. Developing a set of best practices that targets both the commonalities across all generations of learners and the differences between each generation will help instructors facilitate a successful learning experience.

Discussion Questions and Answers
1. Not all learners are comfortable with technology. Based on what you have learned about generational differences, what steps can you take ahead of time to plan for this?

      Understanding the characteristics of the five generations will help to adapt training to be more engaging by providing different options for learning.
2. What are some strategies that you can employ to cater to the different generations of learners in your classes?

      Strategies:

   – Have learners work through information in such a way that they are solving a problem and learning at the same time

- Offer more than one option for delivering content (workbooks, hands-on practice in a playground environment, Flipped Classroom Approach)
- Multitasking, Providing Visual cues with formatting and emphasizing key points
- Reflection to take time out to reflect or process information learned
- Interactive Group activities
- Technology based instruction

3. How can awareness of generational learning perspectives help build more robust learning events?

   The goal of multi-generational training is to encourage commitment from each generation of learners from the instructor's perspectives to focusing on what is important to the learner. Generational awareness can help instructors achieve that goal by being aware of the traits associated with each generation. With generational awareness, instructors can utilize different techniques to enhance the learning environment.

References

1. Lowell VL, Morris J. Leading changes to professional training in the multigenerational office: generational attitudes and preferences toward learning and technology. Perform Improv Q. 2019;32(2):111–35. https://doi.org/10.1002/piq.21290.
2. Marco. Generations in the workplace: Who are they? 2017. Retrieved November 26, 2021 from https://generationsandlearning.wordpress.com/2017/12/04/generations-in-the-workplace-who-are-they/.
3. Dziuban C, Moskal P, Hartman J. Higher education, blended learning and generations: Knowledge is power-no more. Research Initiative for Teaching Effectiveness, LIB. 118, University of Central Florida; 2004.
4. Knight MH. Generational learning style preferences based on computer-based healthcare training. Ph.D., Chapman University; 2016
5. Shatto B, Erwin K. Teaching millennials and generation Z: bridging the generational divide. Creative Nursing. 2017;23(1):24–8. https://doi.org/10.1891/1078-4535.23.1.24.
6. Jones MG, Harmon SW, O'Grady-Jones MK. Developing the digital mind: Challenges and solutions in teaching and learning. Teacher Educ J South Carolina. 2005;2004:17–24.
7. Brown B, ERIC Clearinghouse on Adult Career and Vocational Education. New learning strategies for generation X. ERIC Digest No 184; 1997
8. Driscoll MP, ERIC Clearinghouse on Information and Technology. How people learn (and what technology might have to do with it). ERIC Digest; 2002.
9. Beth A. Longenecker, Teaching Across Generations, Midwestern University, https://www.aacom.org/docs/default-source/2016-Annual-Conference/teaching_across_generations.pdf?sfvrsn=2.
10. Eyler J, Giles D, Schmiede A. A practitioners guide to reflection in service-learning: student voices and reflections. Vanderbilt University Press; 1996.
11. https://www.bluebeyondconsulting.com/thoughtleadership/generational-learning-differences-myth-truth/.
12. Holyoke L, Larson E. Engaging the adult learner generational mix. J Adult Educ. 2009;38(1):12–21.

13. Andriotis N. What is microlearning: a complete guide for beginners. eLearning Industry. 2018; Accessed November 26 2021 from https://elearningindustry.com/what-is-microlearning-benefits-best-practices
14. Soh Y. Bite-sized learning vs. microlearning: are they one in the same? 2017. Retrieved November 26, 2021 from https://elearningindustry.com/bite-sized-learning-vs-micro-learning-are-same

Kathleen Mandato is the Director of Epic Training & Delivery and the Administrative/Nursing Fellowship Program at Vanderbilt University Medical Center. She has worked in the field of training and organizational development for the last 27 years; 10 years in telecommunications, and seventeen years in the healthcare industry. Kathleen has an MBA and a PhD in Education with a specialization in Training & Performance Improvement. She is a registered corporate coach and is Epic Software certified in the Cadence application. Kathleen also teaches healthcare related undergraduate/graduate classes as an Adjunct Professor at Trevecca Nazarene and Cumberland Universities.

Chapter 7
Training Models

Deborah Lewis and Brenda Kulhanek

Growth and Comfort do not Coexist—Ginni Rometty

Abstract Training models provide the guidelines and process steps that can help organize and streamline training development. Several training models have been developed, and while the models have some similarities, they differ in both the focus of the model and the use of the model in development of training. This chapter will focus on three widely used training models: Merrill's five principles for instructional design, Gagne's nine events of instruction, and the ADDIE model. Merrill's five principles for instructional design provide a problem-based model and address the learners' current phase of learning, enabling learners to solve real-life issues. Gagne's nine events of instruction focus on producing successful training through the design and delivery of the instructional content intended to engage learners and increase the success of learning outcomes. The ADDIE model is focused on the process of developing training from start to finish. An overview of each training framework will include application of each framework through practice examples.

Keywords ADDIE · Gagne · Merrill · Training model

D. Lewis (✉)
Doctoral Program, College of Nursing, Walden University, Minneapolis, MN, USA

B. Kulhanek
School of Nursing, Vanderbilt University, Nashville, TN, USA

© The Author(s), under exclusive license to Springer Nature
Switzerland AG 2022
B. Kulhanek, K. Mandato (eds.), *Healthcare Technology Training*, Health
Informatics, https://doi.org/10.1007/978-3-031-10322-3_7

Learning Objectives
1. Verbalize the importance of using a training model to support the production of training.
2. Describe three key training models.
3. Select the best training model to support individual training program development.

The Importance of Using a Training Model

Ryan was new to the training and education team and was excited to get to work. His first project was to develop training for nurses so that they could use a new tool being implemented within the EHR. To get started, he learned all about the new tool and how it functioned within the EHR. As he learned, he captured screen shots of the EHR and the new tool and started to create an eLearning module. After 2 weeks of work, he implemented the new training to all nurses across the hospital. Within 2 hours, Ryan was getting irate emails and phone calls from nurses who had been assigned the new training module. Some nurses complained that they did not use this tool in their specialty area, others used a different workflow than that presented in the training, a few nurses did not possess the foundational technical skills to use the new tool and needed more training, and another group of nurses already used a tool very similar to what was being implemented and did not feel that they needed training.

Why Use a Training Model?

Designing and developing training is a complex process that involves many different stakeholders and considerations. As seen in the story above, although Ryan probably developed a wonderful training program, he missed a few key elements that detracted from the success of the training effort and may have ultimately negatively impacted the adoption of the new functionality for learners who were frustrated by the training. Is it possible to ensure that training is effective and accepted from the start? Training models provide the guidelines and process steps that can help to organize and streamline the production of training. Although Ryan may have created a new training course in record time, when all of the adjustments and revisions of the course were completed, the design and development of the course may not have been as efficient as it could have been.

A Comparison of Training Models

Multiple training models and theories have been developed and used over the last few decades. While the models have some similarities, they differ in both the focus of the model and the processes used within each model. Merrill's *Principles of*

Instruction [1] focuses primarily on the design of the training plan to maximize learner engagement. Gagne's *Nine Events of Instruction* [2] outlines the conditions within the learning environment and delivery structure that are necessary for learning to occur. The ADDIE model is focused primarily on the entire process of developing training from start to finish [3]. The ADDIE model will be discussed briefly in this chapter and the specifics of each step in the ADDIE model will be elaborated in subsequent chapters.

Training is a labor-intensive process and successful outcomes of training are bolstered when an organization uses one or more established training models to plan, structure, and design the training. This section will present a training content model, a training delivery model, and a training development model (Table 7.1).

Merrill's Principles

Rather than an instructional design and development model, Merrill's principles encompass an instructional approach to training that contains common elements found in many design theories and models. Merrill proposed that when training is designed, it should align with five principles. These common principles are the foundation of effective and efficient instruction, and possess some similarities to the adult learning framework. The five principles of instruction are (1) the learner is best engaged when solving problems found in the real world (2) a foundation of existing knowledge should be utilized when adding new knowledge (3) learning is reinforced when the learner can see new knowledge demonstrated (4) the learner must be able to apply the new knowledge, and (5) the learner must integrate new knowledge into their own world [1].

Merrill's first principle states that when learning is designed to be focused on a real-life problem, all aspects of the issue should be combined into the instruction in the form of a real-world task. Combining all topics related to an issue can avoid the

Table 7.1 Training models

Instructional model	Description
Merrill's first principles of instruction	Merrill's First Principles of Instruction identifies five different instructional design principles. This model suggests that training should be centered on real-world issues. A 4-phase cycle includes the learners' prior knowledge, demonstration of new knowledge to the learner, makes students application of new knowledge, and integration of the new knowledge [4]
Gagne's nine events of instruction	Gagne's Nine Events of Instruction are training events that should be used to support success in learning [5]. These events are described fully in the section below. Gagné was instrumental in applying this instructional model to computer and multimedia learning
The ADDIE model	ADDIE remains one of the most popular training models. The model includes 5 phases or steps that guide the training developer. These steps include analysis, design, development, implementation and evaluation [6]

impact of learning each topic in isolation from other related topics. A real-world task can be a simulation, a case study, or an explanation of the problem. Effective instruction begins with showing or presenting to the learner the bigger picture of the entire process in the training content so that they can reference what they are learning in the context of the whole. Within the process of solving the real-world problem, learning activities should progress from the least complex to the most complex. In this process the learner's skills can develop to the point where they can manage more complex processes.

Using Merrill's second principle, when new information or processes are introduced, it is important to relate the new knowledge to existing knowledge so that a foundation of familiarity is developed. During the process the instructor may present examples of prior knowledge that are related to the new concepts, and the learners may be asked to identify these relationships, or share prior knowledge and experience that is related to the new knowledge. At times it may be necessary for the instructor to provide new connections when the concepts being presented do not relate to any existing foundations of experience for the learner.

Demonstration of new knowledge or skills allows the learner to visualize new processes and to observe behaviors to model, as seen in the third of Merrill's principles. The most effective demonstration of new knowledge and skills allows the learner to relate the new knowledge or skill to the overall real-world problem. Demonstrations that are not aligned with a real-world application or problem may decrease the efficiency of learning and contribute to cognitive overload.

The fourth of Merrill's principles involves provision of practice opportunities for learners. The goal of learner practice is for the instructor to coach the learner from dependency to successful navigation of complex problems. Scaffolding can be used to slowly decrease instructor support while increasing the complexity of the practice activities, thus building up knowledge, skill, and repetition to increase competency.

Finally, the fifth principle proposed by Merrill states that the integration phase of learning is achieved in training when learners are able to transfer what they have learned into their own real-life situations. Ultimately, within and after the integration phase, learners should be able to synthesize their ability to address the real-life problem presented in training into addressing similar real-life problems, or utilizing innovation to continue learning.

Merrill's five principles for instructional design provides a model that can guide developers of training to create effective learning that engages learners and produces learning outcomes that enable learners to solve real-life issues.

Gagne's Nine Events

Gagne developed a model in 1965 that outlined the conditions that need to be present for learning to occur. Based on his observations, Gagne developed a nine-step process that is intended to increase the success of learning outcomes by enabling the right conditions for learning. The events are designed to occur in sequence and can be used to create effective eLearning or any other type of learning event.

The first four steps of Gagne's model state that the learning event must begin by gaining the learner's attention and engagement in the training that is to occur. This can be done through group activities, ice-breakers, or a thought-provoking question. When the attention of the learner has been obtained, the second step is to inform the learner of the intended outcome of the training. This explanation may include some discussion of the skills and knowledge that will be needed to obtain the learning outcome. Similar to Merrill's Principles, the third event in Gagne's model is training that should incorporate the existing knowledge and experiences of the learner to provide a foundation for new learning. Step four also aligns with Merrill's Principles by presenting the content or demonstrating a new process in a step by step manner. A second demonstration helps to solidify learning by providing more detail and allowing for discussion and questions.

Event five of the nine events of instruction is designed to help learners encode new knowledge by offering tools and activities that help move information from short-term memory to long-term memory, where it can be retrieved when needed. The sixth event in the Gagne model is introduced after a short break and provides the opportunity for learners to demonstrate what they have learned. In this event learners are paired with each other to demonstrate and assist each other with learning. Step seven is incorporated into step six, so that learners obtain feedback on their performance as they are practicing the new skill or knowledge they have learned.

Gagne's eighth step reinforces new learning as the students perform their new skills independently, guided by an evaluation instrument such as a rubric or checklist. Finally, learning is solidified so that it is retained and is transferable to other situations by including a summary session at the conclusion of the training activity. During the summary session learners are able to ask questions, perform their new knowledge and skills in a real-world environment, and engage in activities that repeat the use of the new knowledge and skills to prevent decay of learning [2].

The ADDIE Model

The term ADDIE is an acronym for analysis, design, development, implementation, and evaluation [6, 7]. The majority of instructional designers use the ADDIE Model or at least a variation to serve as a basis for their work. The advantage of using the ADDIE Model is often cited due to its ease and simplicity that follows a systematic structure. Xing [8] notes that the ADDIE model contributes to superior learning outcomes. In the graphic below (Fig. 7.1) evaluation is central because it occurs throughout the process, first as formative evaluation in the analysis, design and development stages, and as summative evaluation after implementation.

Fig. 7.1 ADDIE model

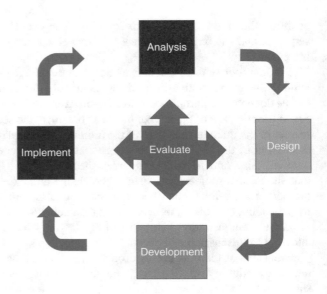

Analysis

The *analysis* phase is the A in the ADDIE model and acts as the base that precedes all other phases of the model. During this phase the training goals and objectives are determined, needs assessments are completed, and organizational support and resources are established. If problems are identified, then the analysis phase allows time to define the given problem or issue in order to formulate feasible solutions. This is also the time to ensure employee readiness for training [6, 7, 9, 10].

Design

The *design* phase continues the groundwork put in place in the Analysis phase and enables the design of training strategies to achieve the established instructional goals. The trainer and the team will create the initial training that consists of the objectives and evaluation components. The design process may also include creating program plans and other plans for complementary training materials [6, 7, 9, 10].

Development

The *development* phase builds on the work completed in both the analysis and design phases. The purpose of this phase is to generate training materials, plans, and supporting documentation. This is also be the time to seek professional development hours to support professional participants, professional development hours, or continuing education hours, are seen as a motivator to engage participation. The development phase is also a chance to test or pilot the training in order to detect deficiencies and apply needed modifications. While informal formative feedback should have occurred in the initial phases, the development phase requires more a more formal approach to formative feedback to ensure that the training materials will meet the expectations of the stakeholders and the established training needs [6, 7, 9, 10].

Implementation

The *implementation* phase refers to the actual delivery of the training to the target group. The training may be delivered in any format. Trainers themselves may need to be trained in this phase to ensure consistent delivery of the training content [6, 7, 9, 10].

Evaluation

Evaluation of the effectiveness of the training takes place throughout the instructional design process and measures the degree of effectiveness and efficiency of instruction. The *evaluation* stage can be carried out throughout the duration of the design process and can be formative or summative. The major evaluation components may require training designers to utilize different evaluation methods, depending on the stage of the project or program. In the analysis phase, evaluation methods are used to review and validate information collected. In the design phase, objectives and strategies are evaluated. In the development stage the training is reviewed, and feedback is provided to ensure that the training plan meets the goals and objectives established for the program. After implementation, summative evaluation consists of measuring participant outcomes related to the learning objectives. Participant satisfaction with the training is also measured at this point [6, 7, 9, 10].

Summary

Training is designed and implemented to address identified gaps in knowledge or skills within an organization. Although the time needed to develop training can vary, based on the complexity of the project, overall the creation of training can be time-consuming. On average, 174 hours of development time are needed to produce 1 hour of classroom training, and 136 hours of development time are needed to create 1 hour of virtual training [11]. The use of established models to create the most effective training content, delivered in the appropriate manner, and developed using a streamlined process employed by organizations throughout the world can increase the likelihood that training will effectively address the identified gaps in knowledge and skills that prompted a training project.

Discussion Questions and Answers

1. What types of activities are used in Gagne's model to ensure that learning occurs?

    (a) Gain the learner's attention through activities, ice-breakers, and discussion questions
    (b) Inform the learners of the intended outcome of the training
    (c) Use existing knowledge and experience as the foundation for new learning
    (d) Use a step-by-step process to present information or to demonstrate
    (e) Include activities that help new information move from short-term to long-term memory
    (f) Provide a break and then have learners demonstrate their new knowledge
    (g) Pair learners to demonstrate what they have learned and provide feedback
    (h) Allow learners to practice independently with a rubric or checklist
    (i) Include a summary session and encourage questions

2. In what ways does Merrill's five principles of learning align with the adult learning framework?

    (a) Principle 1: the learner is best engaged when solving problems in the real world aligns with the adult learning principle of Adults learn best when information is presented or aligned with the context of life or life situations, and The learner wants to know why learning is necessary before investing the time and energy into pursuing learning
    (b) Principle 2: build new knowledge on the foundation of existing knowledge aligns with the adult learning principle of Adults have a great volume of life experience and appreciate learning experiences that acknowledge the value of their past experiences.
    (c) Principle 5: the learner must integrate new knowledge into their own world Aligns with the adult learning principle that adults seek to learn those things that will prepare them for situations or tasks that are imminent; and seek learning that will help them progress in life or accomplish tasks more readily.

3. Why is it important for learners to solve real-world problems when learning?

    (a) Adult learners best engage when learning is directly related to their real world and shows them the big picture

4. In what ways is evaluation conducted in each of the five steps in the ADDIE model?

    (a) Analysis- needs assessment provides the foundation for evaluation of the needs and basis of the learning project
    (b) Design- formative evaluation is used to improve the design of the learning activity
    (c) Development- formative evaluation is used to review and critique the developed learning content for updates and improvements
    (d) Implementation- formative and summative evaluation are collected. Formative evaluation looks at learner response to learning and summa-

tive evaluation explores how well the learning audience learned the information

(e) Evaluation- summative evaluation explore the entire project and seeks to answer the question of whether learning outcomes were met.

References

1. Merrill MD. First principles of instruction. Educ Technol Res Dev. 2002;50(3):43–59. https://doi.org/10.1007/bf02505024.
2. Chen JJ, Johannesmeyer HJ. Gagne's 9 events of instruction with active learning: teaching student pharmacists how to measure blood pressure. J Pharm Pract. 2021;34(3):407–16. https://doi.org/10.1177/0897190019875610.
3. Allen WC. Overview and evolution of the ADDIE training system. Adv Dev Hum Resour. 2006;8(4):430.
4. Merrill MD. First principles of instruction: identifying and designing effective, efficient, and engaging instruction. Association for Educational Communications and Technology; 2020.
5. Gagné RM, Wager WW, Golas KC, Keller JM, Russell JD. Principles of instructional design. 5th ed; 2005. Cengage Learning
6. Branch RM. Instructional design: the ADDIE approach. Springer; 2014.
7. Kurt, S. (2021). ADDIE model: Instructional design. *Educational Technology*. https://educationaltechnology.net/the-addie-model-instructional-design/
8. Xing QY. Application of ADDIE model in instructional design of structural mechanics course. In: *DEStech transactions on social science, education and human science*, (ESEM); 2018. https://doi.org/10.12783/dtssehs/esem2018/23914.
9. Hodell C. The basics of ISD revisited. American Society for Training and Development; 2010.
10. Usta ND, Güntepe ET. Pre-service teachers' material development process based on the ADDIE model: E-book design. J Educ Training Stud. 2017;5(12):199. https://doi.org/10.11114/jets.v5i12.2820.
11. Defelice R. How long does it take to develop training? New questions, new answers. ATD: Association for Talent Development; 2021. https://www.td.org/insights/how-long-does-it-take-to-develop-training-new-question-new-answers

Deborah Lewis Over the course of my faculty career, I have had extensive on-campus and online teaching experience in both undergraduate and graduate programs. I have had experience in building new nursing informatics programs as a faculty developer, member of the leadership team and as an external consultant. I have provided coordination, and teaching to online MSN, DNP and PhD in Nursing programs. My scholarship has included NIH grant funding, publications and presentations in consumer health and chronic illness.

Brenda Kulhanek is an associate professor at the Vanderbilt University School of Nursing and has a history of leadership in both informatics and clinical education. Dr. Kulhanek holds a PhD from Capella University and a DNP from Walden University. She is board certified in nursing informatics, nursing professional development, and executive leadership. Her publications include informatics textbook chapters and multiple informatics articles. She recently participated in the Scope & Standards for Nursing Informatics publication. She teaches informatics at the master's and doctoral levels and has a particular interest in strengthening nursing through nursing informatics education, and the integration of informatics into practice to support improvement of patient outcomes.

Chapter 8
Developing a Training Needs Assessment

Kathleen Mandato

Abstract A Training Needs Assessment is an essential component that helps direct the efforts of the training professional on how to develop a training program that provides the right information to the right people at the right time in the right way. A training needs assessment can identify gaps in performance that lead to helpful recommendations of what to include in the final training solution. It is critical that learners' needs are evaluated prior to the start of training, and in this chapter, the steps of a training needs assessment, along with the purpose of each step, are presented.

Keywords Learning needs assessment · Analysis · ADDIE model · Gaps · Root cause · Primary leader stakeholder (PLS) · Organizational drivers · Training solution

> **Pearls of Wisdom**
> *When it comes to health information technology training, there always seem to be varying levels of knowledge based on learner experiences and roles. A best practice that can be employed with any technology training is to provide a walk-through of a general workflow while the functionality of the system is being explained. However, it is not possible to walk through every specific workflow for every department present at the training. There would not be enough time to go through all of the workflows, and from a learner perspective it would not be engaging to have learners sitting through training that does not directly apply to them. Instead, having learners understand how to work in the system, based on a general workflow, will provide them the foundation that is needed to understand how to navigate through the system and*

K. Mandato (✉)
Epic Training and Delivery and Administrative/Nursing Fellowship Program, Vanderbilt University Medical Center, Nashville, TN, USA

B. Kulhanek, K. Mandato (eds.), *Healthcare Technology Training*, Health Informatics, https://doi.org/10.1007/978-3-031-10322-3_8

understand the technology. From there, individual departments or units can provide more specific on-the-job training to correspond with the nuances of each area.

A helpful tool for reinforcing training content is to provide a workbook with practice exercises that can be performed in a playground or train environment. Assessing the audience prior to training to understand the different specialties represented will allow the training professional to provide scenarios and exercises that are appropriate for each student in the class. While this may not sound like a formal needs assessment, the results are still aligned with many of the objectives of a needs assessment. Learner demographics are being evaluated as well as roles and skills gaps. When creating training, it is important to remember that there will not always be a level playing field. Today's training professional needs to be agile and have the skills to work on the fly to assess stakeholder needs. Whether it is an in depth needs assessment or a rapid just-in time training session, the key point is that the learners' needs must be considered prior to designing and delivering training.

Introduction: The Purpose

A training needs assessment is a critical component in building a successful training program that meets the needs of the learners. Assessing learners and evaluating the who, what, where, why, and how will aid the training professional in creating the transformation that learners will go through as they participate in the training event [1]. Just like a chef or artist prepares and makes plans before working on their master creations, so too does a training professional utilize a training needs assessment to lay out a plan for what content will be provided and how that content will be packaged to deliver a masterpiece.

Analysis or assessment, whichever term you prefer, is the foundation of every successful training program. The ADDIE model consists of five distinct phases and will be presented in subsequent chapters in more detail. The five phases are assessment, design, development, implementation, and evaluation [2]. During the first phase in the ADDIE model, stakeholders will be identified along with barriers and enablers within the organization. This process will ensure a workable learning environment while exploring characteristics of the learning audience. A training analysis provides key pieces of information that help direct the efforts of the training professional.

A training analysis can highlight gaps in performance as well as provide insight into the organization, job, workplace, and learners [3]. The process of assessing provides the opportunity to look at a situation with a new perspective. During the analysis phase, training professionals ask questions, look for problems, imagine a different state, explore, and develop recommendations. The analysis phase of the ADDIE model, "serves as the investigative prelude that informs, first of all whether a program of instruction is needed, and then if so, what outcome should the program

Table 8.1 Needs assessment template

Structure
Organizational drivers
What competing organizational initiatives are occurring at the same time as your planned learning event?
How might these initiatives impact training?
Performance gap
What are the identified knowledge and skills gaps associated with this change?
What are the expected outcomes of this learning event?
What are the consequences of not addressing the knowledge and skills gaps?
How will learning transfer?
When is the learning needed by?
Leadership
What is the level of leadership awareness of the identified knowledge and skills gaps?
What is the level of leadership support for this project?
Is there a primary leader stakeholder?
Culture
Communication
What are the communication channels in the organization?
Who is responsible for communication?
History
Has your organization experienced major changes in the past?
Were there lessons that were learned from those changes?
Current/anticipated drivers for change:
Current/anticipated barriers to change:
Learners
Demographics
Disciplines and specialties of learners
Average skill levels with technology
Attitudes towards change

produce" [4, p. 1]. The following template (Table 8.1) will be discussed section by section and is provided for reference.

Performance Gap

The first part of a needs assessment is to identify the gaps in performance. This step will help determine the overall nature of the problem and potentially the pathway to a solution. Sometimes, after asking questions, it is determined that the identified problem is not related to knowledge or skills, but rather remembering key pieces of a workflow. In this case, a visual reminder or job aide may be in order. Problems that arise may not always be due to training or knowledge gaps. However, training is almost always presented as the solution to any identified issue. Therefore, it is important to ask targeted questions to determine the causes of performance problems or the barriers to optimal performance.

As information is gathered, a set of key questions can be used to help to identify the root cause of a performance problem:

- What are the identified knowledge and skills gaps associated with this change?
- What are the expected outcomes of this learning event?
- What are the consequences of not addressing the knowledge and skills gaps?
- How will learning transfer?
- When is the learning needed by?

These questions will provide a good foundation for determining the cause of the performance problem and if the situation warrants mobilizing the resources needed to create a training solution. As mentioned earlier, sometimes the problems identified are related to the environment, organization, or learner motivation and morale instead of a knowledge gap. Taking the time to properly investigate the situation can provide much needed information for determining the right solution to the problem.

Collecting needs assessment information can be performed in different ways based on time availability and the audience that is providing the information. When determining gaps in performance, the following suggested tools and techniques should be considered:

- Review key performance indicators or dashboards
- Administer learner assessments or quizzes to evaluate knowledge
- Conduct observations
- Interview or survey learners or key stakeholders

Once the gap or gaps are identified, the next step is to determine the desired state. Often, stakeholders already have an idea of what the desired state should be and other times this information must be determined based on an in-depth evaluation of the situation. An important question to consider as the expected outcomes are compiled and reviewed is to understand the extent of the consequences for not addressing the knowledge or skills gap. Asking this question will highlight the importance of the solution and drive organizational commitment and awareness.

At this stage, based on the solution recommended, the choice of how learning will take place may become evident. Gathering initial details regarding the format of the training (online, face-to-face, self-learning, etc.) as well as the expected timeline will help inform and prepare the training professional to work through the next two steps in the ADDIE process, design and develop.

Leadership

Implementing a change or transformation within an organization requires leadership support and commitment. Leaders must be supportive of moving forward with a particular training program and committed to ensuring that the training program receives organizational priority. Having sound leadership in place at all levels to help support the mission and drive accountability toward the completion of the training program is essential in achieving successful results. One of the ways that this can be accomplished is by securing a primary leader stakeholder who can be the champion among other leaders.

The primary leader stakeholder (PLS) can pave the way for leadership alignment in how the training program will be executed and communicated across the organization. The PLS in essence becomes the change agent, articulating the changes needed as well as the reasons and solutions behind the change. In addition, the PLS reinforces accountability with other leaders, which enables consistency and a shared mission. In most cases the PLS is a member of the executive team and well-established within the hierarchy of the organization. Depending on the scope and size of the training implementation, the leadership role may vary. In some cases, based on the change, a mid-level manager or director can assume this role effectively. More information on organizational and leadership commitment and awareness can be found in Chap. 3.

Organizational Drivers

As described early in this chapter, there is usually a root cause that drives organizational change or elevates the need for implementing a training solution. This could be the implementation of a new software product or an associated upgrade, an acquisition of an organization, or establishing a portfolio of new services. Whatever the case may be, timing is everything! It is important to evaluate the landscape and determine if there are competing priorities that could jeopardize a planned learning event. Typically, departments or units must plan ahead and carefully work through training events and schedules to prevent staffing issues. If there is more than one competing priority, this could cause some areas to be overwhelmed and prevent learners from completing required training within the specified timeframe. Even worse, failure to assess for competing projects could cause the planned learning event to take a backseat to another project that has been deemed a higher priority. If learners feel pressured to complete too many assignments or responsibilities, they may not benefit fully from the targeted training solution as their attention is divided between multiple changes and priorities.

Culture

Communication

Good communication is critical in creating awareness and accountability with learners. When the communication or message is not clear, people are more likely to come up with their own interpretation of what is needed. Having a clear communication plan established will help to promote understanding and successful completion of learning events.

The first step in creating a clear communication path is to have someone designated to lead the communication effort. Typically, organizations have a communication manager or coordinator who is responsible for communicating key initiatives out to the organization through different venues such as a newsletter or email. Supplying detailed information to be communicated that includes clear deadlines will help to get the word out to all the right people and to the designated staff scheduled to receive the training. Utilizing an established communication process will ensure that the message is received by everyone needed without unintentionally missing a key stakeholder or group of people. Communication departments and managers typically have a current list of employees to ensure that everyone receives proper communication. Messages coming from a formal communication source are also recognized as having the authority and support of leaders such that learners and other staff take the communication seriously.

The person charged with overseeing the communication, or a designee, should work with different representatives in the organization and provide them a consistent and clear draft of what needs to be distributed. There may be communication protocols in place that require leaders to cascade messages down to their staff. Therefore, leadership commitment is important. Ideally, the PLS would send out a mass communication highlighting the importance of the learning event to everyone. From there, specific communication outlining details of the learning event such as when and how to engage in the learning event would be sent to individual leaders who could then cascade it down to their staff.

Learning events can also be administered through a learning management system (LMS). Individual assignments can be made within the LMS and sent directly to the learner. This method usually works very well when you are certain that a designated group needs the training. When using this method for a larger group of learners, there is a chance that some learners may be assigned a new learning module that they do not need because they have recently changed job roles. For these learners, being assigned unnecessary learning modules can be stressful and upsetting. Staff may not understand why they received the learning assignment and can become agitated with the process because the learning does not pertain to them.

It is important to avoid incorrect learning assignments in the LMS as you begin to assign training. Unless you know for sure who the learning audience should be, using the typical process of assigning learning in an LMS based on job codes or targeting a larger group based on role is not a good idea. If there is doubt, relying on supervisors or managers to assign or communicate the training to their direct reports will eliminate confusion and ensure that the training is being delivered to the appropriate staff.

History

An important part of the assessment process is associated with the culture of the organization. At any given time, the organization may or may not be ready to accept another change. Depending on the size and scope of the training event, assessing where the organization is in terms of being ready to accept another change can make a difference to the success of the learning event. Following are some basic questions that can be asked to determine readiness based on the history of change within the organization:

- Has your organization experienced major changes in the past?
- Were there lessons learned from those changes?
- What are the current and anticipated drivers for change?
- What are the current and anticipated barriers to change?

Understanding what worked well with recent changes will help drive best practices for future change. Likewise, analysis of anticipated barriers can promote awareness and enhanced efforts to provide additional assurances that can alleviate future concerns. The ability to predict certain reactions from groups, based on past history, will be valuable in evaluating an organization's capacity for change.

Learners

Demographics

In order to have a full picture of the group or population that you are targeting for a learning event, it is critical to evaluate their demographics. Understanding demographic characteristics can help inform the format for content design and delivery of training. In this case, demographics refers to the specialty or discipline of the learners. The learning professional needs to determine if all learners perform the same job function, the level of their technical proficiency, the age range of the learners, and the generational spread. Asking these questions will help the learning professional fine-tune the array of content needed. If there are any performance concerns or noted resistance towards a particular change seen in the learner population, having that knowledge will provide a realistic picture of what to expect and how to prepare for it. Being prepared ahead of time will save a lot of time and frustration on the part of the learner and the learning professional.

Stakeholders

Stakeholders are people within an organization who are viewed as resources that add value to the organization. Stakeholders are an important part of conducting a needs assessment because they serve as primary sources of information. They have a vested interest in ensuring the success of the project. Stakeholders not only provide feedback about the gap or performance issue, but also have ideas about how to resolve the issue. Stakeholders can be learners, managers, directors, or patients and customers. The most important reason for involving stakeholders is that once they are part of the process, they most often become committed to ensuring successful outcomes for the project or the changes to come.

Benefits

There is no greater goal or benefit than to observe a learner who feels empowered, or to see the look on a learner's face when understanding and knowledge transfer has been achieved. To create an ideal learning environment, a learning needs assessment must be completed. A learning needs assessment can help identify what should be included in a training solution to achieve specific results. The most important factor in this process is the learner. This assessment is not about the trainer or the organization. It is about ensuring that the learners will be able to meet the objectives outlined for the course and have the tools to successfully perform their job. A learning needs assessment can help prioritize training by focusing on critical elements needed by the organization and therefore demonstrate a positive business impact.

Conclusion

Assessment of learning needs is the first step for designing effective learning events. It is not only a process but a powerful strategy that has been proven effective over many decades. A learning needs assessment saves time and resources by ensuring that the right people receive the right training at the right time, with the best possible results. The contents of this chapter have referenced the different sections contained in the assessment template (Table 8.1).

Discussion Questions and Answers
1. Why is performing a training needs assessment a critical component to building successful training?
   A training needs assessment provides the essential information needed by a training professional to determine the who, what, where, and how for laying out a plan for what content will be provided and how that content will be packaged.
2. How does an assessment help highlight gaps in performance?
   As part of the needs assessment, key questions are asked to determine the identified problem or root cause. These questions will provide a good foundation for determining the cause of the problem and if the situation warrants a training solution or other intervention.
3. How does leadership support help drive accountability for successful completion of training?
   Having sound leadership in place at all levels that help support the mission and drive accountability toward the completion of the training program is essential in achieving successful results. Leadership support helps to ensure that the training goals are met and that other leaders understand the importance of the training.

4. What are the necessary steps in creating successful communication for a learning event?

   The necessary steps for creating successful communication for a learning event are:

   - clear communication plan with a designated person to lead the effort
   - the designated communication person should work with different representatives in the organization and provide them a consistent and clear draft of what needs to be communicated to their staff
   - send LMS communications directly to the learner and ensure that you are targeting the correct staff for the appropriate learning module

5. What is the role of the stakeholder in a needs assessment?

   Stakeholders are an important part of conducting a needs assessment because they serve as primary sources of information. They have a vested interest in ensuring the success of the project. Stakeholders not only provide feedback about the gap or performance issue, but also have ideas about how to resolve the issue. Stakeholders can be learners, managers, directors, or patients and customers. They become committed to ensuring successful outcomes for the project or changes to come.

References

1. Stolovitch HD, Keeps EJ, Rossett A, editors. Analysis for human performance technology. Jossey-Bass/Pfeiffer; 1999.
2. Ritzhaupt A, Covello S. ADDIE explained. Granite State College: Pressbooks; 2022. Retrieved November 26, 2021 from https://granite.pressbooks.pub/addie-explained/.
3. Rossett A. Knowledge management meets analysis. Training Develop. 1999;53(5):62–9.
4. Nichols J, Walsh S, Yaylaci M. Analysis. Granite State College: Pressbooks; n.d. Retrieved November 26, 2021 from https://granite.pressbooks.pub/addie-explained/chapter/analysis/.

Kathleen Mandato is the Director of Epic Training & Delivery and the Administrative/Nursing Fellowship Program at Vanderbilt University Medical Center. She has worked in the field of training and organizational development for the last 27 years; 10 years in telecommunications, and 17 years in the healthcare industry. Kathleen has an MBA and a PhD in Education with a specialization in Training & Performance Improvement. She is a registered corporate coach and is Epic Software certified in the Cadence application. Kathleen also teaches healthcare related undergraduate/graduate classes as an Adjunct Professor at Trevecca Nazarene and Cumberland Universities.

Chapter 9
Designing Training for Best Results

Linda Hainlen

Abstract There are many factors involved in improving processes and outcomes in evidence-based HIT training. All these factors converge when it comes time to design training. Traditionally, designing training is all about identifying learning objectives and creating a curriculum to satisfy the learning objectives. However, this chapter is not just about *designing training* but about *designing training for best results* within the healthcare arena.

Keywords Design · Objectives · Taxonomy · Storyboard · Training methods

Learning Objectives
1. Discuss the difference between being an order taker or a value creator.
2. Describe how to begin with the end in mind when starting the design for any HIT training project.
3. Demonstrate writing learning and performance objectives that point their participants to expected performance after learning.
4. Outline the three stages of learning in the learning process.
5. Discuss the elements of various training methods.
6. Create a learning storyboard for HIT design projects.
7. List the 8 steps of design for any HIT project.

L. Hainlen (✉)
Sedona Learning Solutions, Phoenix, AZ, USA

© The Author(s), under exclusive license to Springer Nature
Switzerland AG 2022
B. Kulhanek, K. Mandato (eds.), *Healthcare Technology Training*, Health
Informatics, https://doi.org/10.1007/978-3-031-10322-3_9

103

It was in the news nationally. It was in the news internationally. The wrong dosage of medication was given to five patients at our hospital and three of them died. .. What a dark, dark day for healthcare. When I received the request to train clinicians on a new medication administration process, I worked hard to understand the expected outcomes from the project and really focused on creating stellar learning experiences that addressed the knowledge and skills gaps. Students were passing their assessment during class and I was excited to be part of the solution.

Leadership had agreed that a 90% compliance rate was the goal. When I received a medication compliance report 2 weeks after go-live, it had only reached 66%. What happened? People passed their assessments during class. Why didn't this translate to compliance? Determined to find out, I went to the units and asked nurses to demonstrate that they knew how to use the system as trained. They knew how. When I asked why they were not following what was taught, they replied, "Look, I am really busy, so unless someone tells me I have to pass meds this way, I am not going to."

So where did I fail? I failed when I designed for learning instead of best results.

There are many factors to improving processes and outcomes in evidence-based HIT, and as covered in previous chapters, many of them involve working with other disciplines. All these factors converge when it comes time to designing training. Traditionally, designing training is all about identifying learning objectives and creating a curriculum to satisfy the learning objectives. However, this chapter is not just about *designing training* but about *designing training for best results* within the healthcare arena.

The design process involves making a *blueprint* for the training experience through the selection and creation of measurable objectives, the instructional method, lesson plans that include exercises and interactivity, and evaluation tasks and tools.

Learning Enabler or Value Creator?

An informaticist analyzes and determines how the use of technology can improve patient care. However, a disconnect often exists between the analysis and organizational outcomes. This can lead to an unfortunate pattern: a deficiency in reaching an outcome is identified, a learning course is requested and provided, yet nothing happens and the deficiency remains.

Organizations often ask for a *quick fix* training solution such as an automated electronic presentation or a check box to acknowledge training, but they expect better results than what automated presentations and acknowledgements can typically provide. The organization expects not only that learning will happen, but that learning will be implemented on the job, and that this improvement in performance will then make a measurable difference in key organizational results.

How should an informaticist or learning professional respond, then, when asked to provide training? Andy Lancaster in his book *Driving Performance Through Learning* offers options based on four workplace personas (Fig. 9.1) [1]. *Order takers* would simply design the training based on the request, no questions asked. In contrast, *learning enablers* would design training based on learning objectives and provide participants with knowledge to meet those objectives. *Performance enablers* move beyond supplying knowledge to creating training in which learners apply new knowledge during skill practice.

While each of these three personas design parts of an ideal training solution, the informaticist focused on creating the most effective training will be a *value creator*. Value creators are the most successful at bringing real value to their organizations because their training solutions do not stop with theoretical knowledge or even classroom practice. They follow through with tools to support learners where the actual application happens on the job. So, although a specific training design may be requested, value creators will consider the performance-based results the organization hopes to achieve as they analyze the training need. If they find that the requested design does not align with the desired results, value creators will speak up and help others understand the need for a training project that will truly make it possible for clinicians to achieve the outcomes that are being sought.

Deciding which role you will take in your curriculum design projects will have a definite impact on your results. In today's healthcare climate that is fraught with new clinical challenges, advanced research, staffing shortages and budget cuts, it is more important than ever to move beyond learning to value by designing for true outcomes.

Fig. 9.1 Training personas

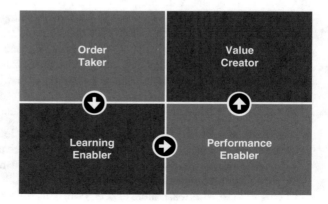

Begin with the End in Mind

Adult learning theory, design models, and analysis have already been explored in previous chapters. Once the analysis is complete (Chap. 8) and an evaluation plan created (Chap. 12), design of the curriculum can begin. But how does curriculum design begin? Stephen R. Covey's advice to *begin with the end in mind* bears repeating here [2]. Informatics can identify many areas of needed improvement, but often must prioritize changes that will be implemented because of time and resource limitations. This prioritization is most easily accomplished by truly understanding the desired *end*, or organizational goals and the desired performance outcomes.

This process first begins during the analysis stage, when the problem statement is combined with associated risks and benefits which lead to the desired outcome. Understanding the business need and desired outcomes is imperative in designing the curriculum and pointing the learner to what is expected of them and why. Typically, the business need for the training project is defined in the analysis stage when the problem statement is combined with associated risks and benefits, which leads to the desired outcome. Once the business need and desired outcome are documented, the behaviors needed to meet the business need can be identified. Once the needed and desired behaviors are documented, gaps in knowledge, skills, and attitude can be identified. Then, and only then, can you begin to design a training intervention. Remember, in academia, learning in and of itself can sometimes be the goal. In HIT training, *achieving results from learning* is the goal.

Point the Learner to Performance with Objectives

Once all the necessary information and data from analysis has been gathered, the first step in designing a training curriculum is to create performance objectives. Well-defined performance objectives provide the training designer with direction for the creation of course materials. They also provide training participants with a clear understanding of what is expected of them at the end of the course, and on the job. Lastly, performance objectives can inform participants of the broader desired business outcomes. This often helps participants to see the *why* for new performance expectations.

A well-defined learning or performance objective contains three parts:

A beginning similar to the following: "At the conclusion of this course, the *participant will be able to*...." (Note that training provides the ability to do a specific task, but until on-the-job application occurs, the learner has not yet had the opportunity to complete the task as part of their work performance. Therefore "being able to" is a reasonable expectation. This objective aligns with a Level 2 evaluation, which is covered in Chap. 12.

Part	Example Content
Beginning	At the conclusion of this course, the participant will be able to
Verb and Noun	correctly document administered cancer medications in the electronic health system
Expected Outcome	so that reimbursement is increased and budget cuts can be avoided

Fig. 9.2 Creating a performance objective

A verb and a noun: Verbs and nouns define what the participant will be able to do after training and typically are verbs associated with Bloom's taxonomy of learning ([3] p. 44 Fig. 9.3).

The expected outcome. This reaches beyond the learning event to the expected outcome, which provides motivation and communicates expectation for the learner's performance on the job. The expected outcome aligns with a Level 3 evaluation, which is addressed in Chap. 12.

This same process can be repeated for any type of learning or performance objective.

A well-designed performance objective can be seen in Fig. 9.2.

The performance objective will guide decisions about what content is delivered during training such as the steps needed to correctly document and cancel medications. The actions that will be evaluated are included in the performance objective, and include what the learner should be able to know or demonstrate at the conclusion of training.

Among the tools available to help create effective performance objectives, Blooms Taxonomy deserves mention. This straightforward model of the learning process was proposed in 1956 by Benjamin Bloom and updated in 2001 ([3] p. 44 Fig. 9.3). Like other taxonomies, Bloom's taxonomy is hierarchical, meaning that learning at the higher levels is dependent on having attained prerequisite knowledge and skills at lower levels.

In Blooms Revised Taxonomy, each level is built on the foundation of obtaining the previous levels, as depicted in Fig. 9.3. The basic premise is:

- Before you can understand a concept, you must *remember* it.
- To apply a concept, you must first *understand* it.
- To evaluate a process, you must have *analyzed* it.
- You must have completed a thorough *evaluation* to *create* an accurate conclusion.

In HIT training, clinicians often come to a learning event with a certain level of basic knowledge, so it is not always necessary to design objectives and material that will step participants through the entire taxonomy. In addition, if an entirely new concept will be addressed in a training event, lower levels can be covered in prerequisite, independent learning to set the stage for higher levels of learning. Table 9.1 contains verbs that correspond with each level of learning that can be used in creating performance objectives.

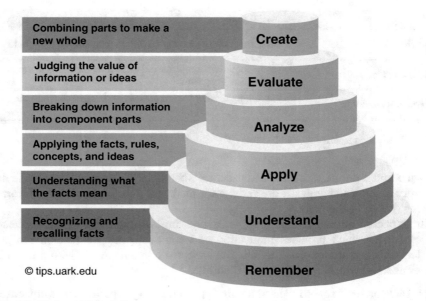

Fig. 9.3 Updated Bloom's Taxonomy

Table 9.1 Taxonomy verbs

Create	Create, combine, compile, modify, organize, reorganize, summarize, devise, design
Evaluate	Evaluate, appraise, compare, conclude, conrast, critique, defgind, interpret, justify, support
Apply	Apply, change, compute, consruct, demonstrate, discover, modify, operate, prepare, produce, show, use
Understand	Convert, define, distinguish, estimate, explain, give an example, interpret, paraphrase, predict, rewrite
Remember	Define, describe, identify, label, list, match, name, outline, recall, recognize, reproduce, select, state

Fig. 9.4 Burch's four
stages of learning

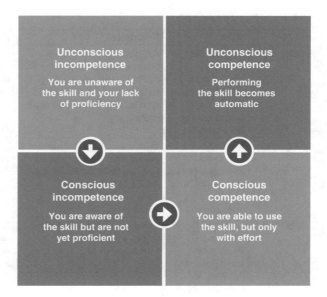

Learning Is a Process, Not an Event: Design for Three Stages of Learning

As outlined with Bloom's Taxonomy, learning is a complex process. This process was also described by Noel Burch in the 1970s, see Fig. 9.4. Burch proposed that learners move through four stages: being unaware of a lack of proficiency, or *unconscious incompetence*, becoming aware, or *conscious incompetence*, being able to perform the skill but only with much thought and effort, *conscious competence*, and finally, performing the skill automatically without effort, or *unconscious competence* [4].

Both Bloom and Burch point to the reality that learning is much more than a single event but a process that moves the learner from incompetence to competence (Table 9.2). Therefore, the design of any program should be broken down into three phases of learning.

For the success of any HIT project it is crucial to ensure the design includes these three stages of learning to ensure outcomes are derived from learning. Clear deliverables for all three stages should be identified. All too often the design only includes the formal learning event which ensures learning happens, but leaves outcomes to chance.

In addition to creating clear deliverables for each stage, the HIT professional should also identify how each stage will be measured and evaluated for effectiveness. As noted in Chap. 12, both formative and summative data should be collected and reviewed early during each stage so adjustments can be made if necessary.

Table 9.2 Three phases of learning

Stage	Name	Description	Examples of interventions
Stage one	Prerequisite learning Unconscious incompetence to the door of conscious incompetence	Any form of prerequisite learning that sets the stage for a formal learning event by making the learner aware of their lack of knowledge and/or proficiency	Online tutorials, communications to the learner and their supervisors, games, staff meeting topics
Stage two	Learning event Conscious incompetence to the door of conscious competence	Where training takes place and participants become able to perform tasks. Should include reinforcement through exercises, role play, and/or simulation	Classroom experience, virtual classroom experience, online tutorial
Stage three	Performance on the job Conscious competence to the door of unconscious competence	Change is difficult and often requires performance to be driven	Just-in-time tools and job aids, social interaction, peer collaboration, manager encouragement and accountability

Workplace Training Methods

Part of the design process is identifying training methods for all three stages of learning. There are many options available, from traditional to more modern technology solutions. In HIT training, the role preferences for training methods can vary greatly. For instance, it is often difficult to get physicians to attend classroom training, but the majority will find time to complete an online tutorial. Many report that they enjoy the fact that they can complete training when they want, where they want, and at the pace they want.

The content of the training also helps determine which training delivery method would be appropriate. When training a large volume of new material, such as a new EHR system, a three stage, blended approach is educationally sound and provides for better outcomes. In this instance, you might consider:

Stage 1: An eLearning tutorial to cover baseline of new information
Stage 2: A shortened classroom experience wherein participants can review content covered in the prerequisite tutorial, practice, and ask questions
Stage 3: Micro-performance support tools combined with preceptor coaching

When a small update to an EHR system is to be trained, a short online tutorial may be sufficient. HIT training methods come in all shapes and sizes, and the variety keeps growing with each passing year. What follows is a simple guide detailing some of the most common methods to help you find the training method that fits your organization's needs [5, 6].

Choosing the Right Training Method

Before choosing a training method, the information obtained during the analysis phase can help guide the choice of delivery method. Informatics gathered during analysis should include the training goals, the target audience, the learning preference of the target audience, available resources, budget and timeline constraints, and how success will be measured. How will you measure success? Once this information has been verified and clarified, the task of selecting the best way to train the learning audience can begin.

Training Method One: Instructor-Led Training (ILT)

Instructor-led training (ILT) refers to training that occurs in a physical or virtual classroom. ILTs are most beneficial for complex content because learners have the option to ask questions directly and receive immediate clarification. ILTs can be further categorized into the following types, as seen in Table 9.3.

Training Method Two: eLearning

eLearning, or online training, has become one of the most widely recognized solutions for training delivery. Online workplace training can include eLearning courses with video tutorials that provide a more visual presentation of the training content. True eLearning is engaging and interactive and not merely the presentation of information through automated presentations. eLearning is relatively inexpensive and reduces need for clinicians to attend classroom training. However, because of these factors eLearning is also sometimes overused.

Training Method Three: Immersive or Experiential Learning

Immersive learning provides learners with an interactive learning environment where it is possible to replicate real-life scenarios or teach particular skills. Methods involving this type of learning can be further categorized as seen in Table 9.4.

Table 9.3 Types of ILT

Face-to-face training	The traditional classroom training method that has been around for quite some time. Lectures, conferences, and seminars are examples of this method
Virtual classroom	Participants can communicate and interact in an online setting, mostly through video conferencing. They can collaborate with the instructor as well as the other learners
Webinar	Learners participate in an online lecture. They can post questions and answer polls. In most cases, learners interact with the instructor and not with fellow learners

Table 9.4 Immersive learning

Simulations	Popular in larger healthcare institution. They provide for a specialized form of immersive learning that focuses on demonstration of skills and allows the learners to make decisions in a risk-free environment and experience the consequences of their actions
Virtual reality (VR)	A form of interactive software that recreates a real-world environment in a 3D virtual space. Participants can learn new skills or practice old ones without worrying about the consequences of failure
Scenario-based interactive video	Allows trainees to change the learning process from passive to active by allowing the learner to make choices that branch to options that meet their learning needs

Table 9.5 Social learning

Mentoring/ Coaching/ Precepting	A semi-structured method of guidance in which the mentor shares their knowledge and experience to help others progress in their skills
Just-in-time performance support	Micro learning, which is short snippets of content, and job aids serve as add-on or refresher information that is available at the point of need. In HIT, the point of need is often at the bedside and needs to be readily available and succinct

Training Method Four: Just-in-Time and Social Learning

Social learning is not a new concept. It happens effortlessly when people communicate with peers about how to perform a task, receive mentoring from a preceptor, or observe other people's actions. Social learning on the job happens frequently but can create unintended results that veer from best practice. Therefore, support for social interactive learning needs to be planned. For instance, preceptors can be trained to use best practices when mentoring learners, supported with just-in-time learning aids micro-learning modules or job aids. Table 9.5 further describes each of these training tools.

Training Method Five: Blended Learning

Blended learning refers to a teaching method that integrates technology and live location-based classroom activities and allows learners to get the best of both online and traditional learning. As seen in Table 9.6, some common types of blended approaches are described.

The Pros and Cons of Training Methods

To help select the most appropriate training method(s) for a project, Table 9.7 lists some pros and cons for each teaching method [7].

Table 9.6 Blended learning

Flipped model	The reverse of traditional classroom teaching where the learners are taught in the class and then given homework. In this model, the learners are provided content before the class. They go through it independently online. During the classroom session, they discuss the content and perform various activities to ensure that they have understood the concepts. Support tools are then supplied at the point of need.
Face-to-face driver model	A chunk of classroom session is replaced with online activities, tutorials, or videos. This model works well for new hire training where the audience is captive, but the facilitator can take advantage of utilizing online tutorials and activities and operate more as a proctor.
Flex model	In this setup, the learners complete most of their courses online with a small portion of in-person activities like drop-in labs on an as-needed basis. This is a flexible model that is often appealing to physicians.

Table 9.7 Training method pros and cons

Method	Pros	Cons
Classroom/ILT	• ILT has a personal touch. The instructors and the learners can interact directly face to face. They can gauge each other's body language and adapt accordingly. • The learners can get immediate answers to questions and clarification on confusing concepts. • Group interactions help learners learn.	• It can be quite expensive to pull clinicians off the floor and may require travel to a specific site. • Classrooms have limited space for participants. • Classroom training creates a lot of logistics in scheduling. • Staffing may have to be augmented to cover for clinicians who are in the classroom. • The speed of the class follows the mean of the participants.
eLearning	• Learners can access learning anytime they want and from anywhere. • Learners can choose their own pace.	• If the target audience is not tech savvy, they may not find computer-based training suitable. • The learners do not have instant face-to-face access to an instructor to ask questions. • May require purchase of an authoring tool and/or a learning management system.
Immersive/ Experiential	• Immersive learning keeps the learners engaged. As a result, they learn better and recall faster. • Since it is a risk-free environment, participants can learn without having to pay a penalty for making mistakes. • The participants are given instant feedback on their actions. That way they know where they've gone wrong and can avoid the behavior in the workplace.	• Creating an immersive learning experience can be cost and time intensive. • If you fail to recreate the relevant job environment completely, the participants may not be able to fully immerse themselves in the situation. • Some platforms need regular updating and maintenance.

(continued)

Table 9.7 (continued)

Method	Pros	Cons
JIT/social	• By tutoring others, clinicians can gain valuable knowledge and skills on their own. • Social learning can help develop a learning community and improve communication and collaboration. • Learners can ask questions and receive answers at the point of need which reduces frustration.	• Social learning can be difficult to control and if proper information is not shared, workarounds are born. • Limited data to show how social learning works for calculating a return.
Blended	• Blended learning provides great flexibility in presenting the content to learners. The complex parts can be presented face-to-face, and the rest can be made available online. • Since modern learners are often surrounded by technology, they remain more engaged when you incorporate technology in learning. • You can reach a higher number of learners with digitized content. • A blended learning approach reduces the classroom teaching time.	• Blended learning methods have a strong dependence on technology. • Learners don't always have high connectivity. When the connection is slow, it may take a long time for the content to download, and they may lose their patience. • If online content is too extensive and not provided in digestible lengths, learners can lose interest and retention of information.

There are many types of activities that can be incorporated in learning methods that will increase engagement of participants that include role play, scenario-based exercises, gaming, and more. Additional training activities are covered further in Chapters 10 and 11 in this textbook.

Creating a Learning Storyboard

A storyboard is a planning document for the development of curriculum. As the name suggests, a storyboard tells the story or creates the framework of a training course. A storyboard is created before the learning deliverables are created and provides a roadmap of how the learning experience will unfold in a step-by-step manner. Once the storyboard has been completed and approved, learning professionals can proceed with course development.

Instructional design principles and adult learning theory should guide the storyboarding process. These principles help to organize and present course content in a way that engages the learner. In addition to developing content for all three phases of learning, the designer should select a delivery method for each phase, consider how to connect with the learner visually, select exercises or learning activities that will promote learner engagement, and include how the learning will be evaluated in both a formative and summative manner.

There are several storyboard software packages available that can be used. Alternatively, a simple computerized text document or spreadsheet can be utilized to create a storyboard. Included in Fig. 9.5 is an example of a storyboarding template created in Microsoft Word.

Steps to Putting the Design Process into Action

The design process touches almost every other part of training development and delivery. As stated at the beginning of this chapter, many factors converge in the design of a training program. A summary of the steps involved, along with where to locate more information about the factors pertaining to each step, is seen in Table 9.8.

In summary, understanding organizational outcomes combined with what is known about the learners' current knowledge, attitude, and behaviors leads to the development of learning objectives and the selection of learning methods that will support the learner through all stages of acquiring competency in using HIT on the job. After all information has been collected, the plan to accomplish the learning outcomes, the curriculum design, is documented on the storyboard. A carefully constructed storyboard will guide the development and delivery of all learning materials. It will ensure that your training project leads participants through all stages of learning and results in a change in behavior that garners results for every HIT training project.

Discussion Questions
1. In what ways is it important to be a value creator rather than an order taker?
2. Why is important to start an HIT training project with the end in mind?
3. What is the difference between learning objectives and performance (or outcomes) objectives?
4. What are three benefits of using a storyboard when designing instruction?
5. What are the three stages of learning in the learning process?

Discussion Questions and Answers
1. Why is performing a training needs assessment a critical component to building successful training?
   This process first begins during the analysis stage, when the problem statement is combined with associated risks and benefits which lead to the desired outcome. Understanding the business need and desired outcomes is imperative

Project Name:			
Date:	Author:	Version:	Approval:
Problem Statement:		Desired Outcomes:	
Behaviors Needed		Learning Gaps to be Addressed	
1. 2. 3.		1. 2. 3.	
Learning/Performance Objectives			
1. 2. 3.			

Phase 1 – Prerequisite Learning*			
Learning Objective 1:			
Task	Content	Supporting Activities/Visuals	Evaluation Methods
Task 1			Formative:
Task 2			Summative:
Learning Objective 2:			
Task	Content	Supporting Activities/Visual	Evaluation Methods
Task 1			Formative:
Task 2			Summative:

Phase 2 – Learning Event*			
Learning Objective 1:			
Task	Content	Supporting Activities/Visuals	Evaluation Methods
Task 1			Formative:
Task 2			Summative:
Learning Objective 2:			
Task	Content	Supporting Activities/Visual	Evaluation Methods
Task 1			Formative:
Task 2			Summative:

Phase 3–Performance Support			
Behavior	How will behavior be driven?	Supporting Tool(s)/Delivery Method	Content if Applicable
Behavior 1	Support: Accountability:		
Behavior 2	Support: Accountability:		
Behavior 2	Support: Accountability:		

* If the learning method includes eLearning, you will want to add a column for slide number, branching, etc.

Fig. 9.5 The storyboard

Table 9.8 Design input sources

Step:	Supporting Chapters:
1. Having a clear understanding of the project and expected outcomes. (assessment stage which includes needs analysis, expected outcomes, behaviors needed, learning gaps that need to be addressed, etc.)	Chapter 8: Needs Assessment
2. Reviewing evaluation plan and assessment criteria for inclusion in the design (evaluation planning stage)	Chapter 12: Evaluation Chapter 13: Assessing Competency
3. Defining learning/performance objectives	Chapter 9: Design
4. Creating a storyboard addressing three stages of learning	Chapter 9: Design
5. Selecting a training method for each stage	Chapter 9: Design
6. Selecting a training model and formulating content	Chapter 6: Generational Differences Chapter 7: Training Models and Theories
7. Choosing design elements such as supporting activities and visual aids	Chapter 11: Training Delivery
8. Obtaining approval and handoff to development	Chapter 10: Development

in designing the curriculum and in pointing the learner to what is expected of them and why. Typically, the business need is defined in the analysis stage when the problem statement is combined with associated risks and benefits which leads to the desired outcome. Once the business need and desired outcome are documented, the behaviors needed to meet the business need can be identified. Once needed/desired behaviors are documented, gaps in knowledge/skills/attitude can be identified. Then, and only then, can you begin to design a training intervention.

2. How does an assessment help highlight gaps in performance?

Once needed/desired behaviors are documented, gaps in knowledge/skills/attitude can be identified. Then, and only then, can you begin to design a training intervention.

3. Select a training method and provide the rationale for why that method would be used, including the learner audience.

4. Why does Bloom's taxonomy contain multiple levels of learner performance objectives?

In Blooms Revised Taxonomy, each level is built on a foundation of the previous levels as depicted in Fig. 9.3. The basic premise is:

- Before you can understand a concept, you must *remember* it.
- To apply a concept, you must first *understand* it.
- To evaluate a process, you must have *analyzed* it.

You must have completed a thorough *evaluation* to *create* an accurate conclusion.

Days of the Week Exercise

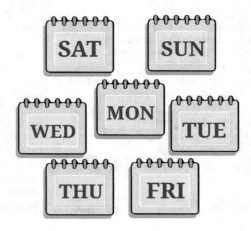

1. Ask students to push their chairs far enough away from their desk to stand up.
2. Tell them, when you say go, to say the days of the week, beginning with Monday, as fast as they can. When they have completed the task, stand up. Repeat instructions and say "go". (They should all stand up at pretty close to the same time)
3. Now, ask them to remain standing and tell them you are going to ask them to complete the exercise in a different way. Ask they if they have any guesses. Typically they will say, "in reverse order".
4. Say "no", I want you to say them in alphabetical order. When they say them in alphabetical order, they may sit down. Go. (You will typically see some students visualizing a job aid in their minds, some will give up, etc.)
5. Now, ask them:

   a. if you gave them a test on the what the days of the week are, would they pass?
   b. If you gave them a test on their alphabetizing skills, would they pass?
   c. If you asked them to say the days of the week in alphabetical order from now on, how easy would it be?**Point: Just because students learn content and can pass a test, does not mean they will implement what they have learned. To obtain performance, support needs to be in place to drive performance—accountability by supervisors, job aids, rewards, etc. Never design for just learning, design for three stages of learning to promote outcomes.**

References

1. Lancaster A. Driving performance through learning: develop employees through effective workplace learning. Kogan Page Limited; 2020.
2. Covey SR. First things first. Simon Schuster; 1994.
3. Anderson LW, Krathwohl DR, editors. A taxonomy for learning, teaching and assessing: a revision of Bloom's taxonomy of educational objectives: Complete edition. Longman; 2001.
4. Burch N. Conscious Competence Theory of learning a new skill: The four stages of competence; 1970. Retrieved September 27, 2021, from https://www.mccc.edu/~lyncha/documents/stagesof competence.pdf.
5. Andriotis N. 5 popular employee training methods for workplace training; 2018. Retrieved September 1, 2021, from https://elearningindustry.com/how-choose-training-methods-for-employees
6. Colman H. 6 training methods in the workplace: Choose the best for your employees; 2019. Retrieved September 1, 2021, from https://www.ispringsolutions.com/blog/training-methods
7. Shabatura J. Using Bloom's Taxonomy to write effective learning objectives; 2013. Retrieved September 1, 2021, from https://tips.uark.edu/using-blooms-taxonomy/

Linda Hainlen is the Director of Business Development at Sedona Learning Solutions, a Kirkpatrick Certified Facilitator, and an international speaker and author. She served as Director of Learning Solutions for IU Health in Indianapolis, IN for 18 years. Linda has over 25 years of proven experience as a training manager and has worked with companies from around the world to improve their effectiveness and achieve measurable outcomes.

Linda has been published several times, including a white paper co-written with Jim Kirkpatrick on the topic of healthcare. Her ATD Infoline on "Designing Informal Learning" made the top 50 best sellers and was translated into 83 languages.

Chapter 10
Developing Training

Kathleen Mandato

Abstract This chapter explores the components that go into developing a fully functional learning experience that aligns with the project plan and learning objectives. During the development phase, the right technology is selected based on evaluation of the learner profile and need. Finding the right balance between training and technology will help to promote better learning engagement.

Keywords Prototype · eLearning · Learning technology · Training development

Learning Outcomes
1. Identify current learning technologies
2. Understand and select the best learning technology for the training need
3. Verbalize the components of the development phase of ADDIE

K. Mandato (✉)
Epic Training and Delivery and Administrative/Nursing Fellowship Program, Vanderbilt University Medical Center, Nashville, TN, USA

B. Kulhanek, K. Mandato (eds.), *Healthcare Technology Training*, Health Informatics, https://doi.org/10.1007/978-3-031-10322-3_10

121

Selecting the Right Technology
The training team spent many hours creating a beautiful eLearning lesson to address the upcoming EHR update. This was the first time the team was using eLearning to deliver training and they were excited to observe the reactions of the nurses to this new time-saving method of training. After a series of planning communications, the training was assigned to all of the nurses through the LMS. After a few weeks, the rate of lesson completion remained very low, despite ongoing communication. Finally, a nurse working in the ICU mentioned in passing that the computers nurses use for patient care do not have sound cards in them, therefore the nurses were not able to view and hear the learning modules between patients. Sometimes the unexpected can derail an otherwise wonderful training plan!

Training and the Right Technology

The right technology can help enhance training and make it more beneficial for learners. Technology can turn everyday training into something interactive and exciting that can be delivered to learners anywhere at any time. The right technology can also be customized to fit the needs of the learners while helping to enhance retention and engagement.

Technology

The human touch may always be needed to train new employees and develop curriculum to meet the needs of the learners. However, at some point, the extent and scope of the audience will require a different approach to maintain the quality and consistency of training across several locations within an organization. There becomes a need to be efficient while maintaining the desired level of engagement with learners. There are also logistical challenges to consider, such as how to distribute training manuals or other training documents. These paper-based items often require regular updates when information changes. The need for a more flexible solution that provides accurate real time information without the associated waste of paper, travel time, and other resources becomes a necessity.

Based on organizational and learner profiles, the training process is shifting from training at a single location to an increase in remote learning as organizations become less centralized. Many employees are now telecommuting because of the recent COVID pandemic. Since in-person learning may not be feasible, it is important to provide alternative options for continuous learning so that learners are able to stay updated on changing regulations or compliance related items. The ability to train in several locations at once without losing anything in translation is the new reality of health care and many other industries. While using hands-on technology for training has been essential in many organizations, new options to learn or enhance skills are becoming more accessible than ever before.

Following the *Design* phase, the *Development* phase of the ADDIE Model consists of course creation when learning professionals begin to develop content, identify, and integrate the content into the technology that is the best solution for the learning event. At this point, learning professionals are following a roadmap, or storyboard, that was created to keep them on track during the *Analysis* and *Design* phases. Learning professionals are guided by the instructional goals of the training project, have established the learning environment and possess a completed learner assessment. The purpose of the *Development* phase is to develop a fully functional learning experience that aligns with the established project plan and learning objectives created in the previous ADDIE phases [1]. Since the content has already been decided upon, during this phase the focus is on organizing the content so that it is ready for implementation.

Drafting and Prototyping

There are three major steps involved in the development phase, drafting and prototyping, producing materials, and testing and evaluating [2].

The drafting and prototyping phase is all about building the learning materials to reflect the design plan. This step involves putting the pieces of content together to produce a draft or *prototype* of the finished product. This prototype will be used to demonstrate the main learning concepts and can be presented to stakeholders for final approval and feedback regarding any changes that may be needed. The prototype is a shorter version of the final product that provides an overall idea of what the final concept will look like when everything is completed. Also included in the prototype should be a short summary of the course plan to ensure understanding of the overall strategy and intent of the learning event [2].

The next phase on the development journey is to produce materials such as the content, lesson plans, exercises, and potentially eLearning materials needed for the learning event. At this point, any technology to be used is developed and integrated into the final product. Often, the technology used for the learning event is selected in the design phase. However, there are important considerations involved in order to evaluate, select, and confirm the right technology for the learning design and purpose. Reflecting on the purpose and learning objectives are key to considering any technology options.

The Learners

It is important that training is accessible to as many learners as possible. Consideration must be given to those learners with disabilities as well as other learners and their ability to have access to training content both at home and at work. Questions to consider include any need for learners to purchase new technology for learning, and the readiness of learners to use technology. The responses to these questions will guide the design of the learning event. Learning professionals must determine if using technology is appropriate for learning the content that is proposed. If the conditions are not aligned for using technology-driven training, then the learning specialist must take steps to ensure that technology driven training is the right course to take [3].

Ease of Use

When it is clear that training delivery through technology is the right course to take, the next step is to select the right technology, if the technology was not determined in the design phase of the project. The selected technology provides the platform needed to deliver the learning content and must be easy to use by both the learner and instructor. Another consideration is to ensure that maintenance and set-up of the technology are simple and straightforward. No matter which vendor is being used, it is important to confirm that there will be support for hardware and software use in case of problems. There have been times when a technology platform provider ceases business, therefore it is important to identify a way to secure the training content and materials produced in case something happens with the vendor. It is also necessary to have design and technical support to help with creating and editing content and to make sure that learners will benefit from the learning technology and that the content is built into the technology in a way that will produce the best learning experience and outcomes [3].

Cost and Time

Time is an important component in the search for the right training media platform. The selected platform must be straightforward and easy enough to use so that there is ample time to develop the content. In addition to the time needed to develop the basic content, the learning professional must determine if there is time to add additional features that are more interactive and encourage engagement to stimulate increased learning. Developing training in a technology platform may be the best solution for the learners and save time for the developers, but the work should be scoped in the project plan to ensure that the selected technology approach will be the better overall solution for the learners and potentially save time for creators. Identification of organizational support and resources for media design is important and will help enhance the final learning product. Based on the content, learning professionals may also consider additional online resources such as literature related to the learning or videos that will help support the learner and encourage more online activity and self-guided exploration.

Interaction

Interaction plays a key role in supporting the learner's ability to process the content that is delivered. Most learners are familiar with the traditional instructor-led classroom format. This format is an efficient way for presenting a large amount of content to a large group of people. This training approach provides a personal touch with the face-to-face model of training, but the large classroom format often lacks interactivity. The classroom method relies on the facilitator to stay engaging and to be creative with different techniques to hold the learners' attention. Creating interactive online training helps keep the learners attentive and involved while allowing them the flexibility to complete their training at their own pace. Depending on the situation and what makes sense for the learner, there are a variety of different technology options that can be employed when the decision is made to use technology as the delivery method.

Training Delivery Methods

Computer-Based Training

Computer-based training (CBT) is a great option that allows for organizations and employees to have more control over the learning process. CBT involves the use of a personal or networked computer for the delivery of training or access to training. CBT can be synchronous or asynchronous, and it can be presented as online, web-based, mobile, and distance learning. The CBT format can be engaging and easily accessed by learners through a smartphone or other device anywhere and anytime. CBT training is structured and linear and the learner follows a specific path to completion of the learning [4]. When taking a CBT approach to training delivery, it is a good idea to explore training technologies and be aware of what is available. Even if an organization decides not to use this method as the primary method for delivering training, the CBT approach can still help enhance current in-person learning platforms. There are several options for different types of CBT and listed in Table 10.1 is a compilation of the different types.

Table 10.1 CBT formats

Format	Description
Text-only	• Self-paced training in text-only with interactive features
CD-ROM	• Already created training programs available to purchase off the shelf
Multimedia	• More robust than just text-based-offers animation, graphics, audio, and video
Virtual reality	• Three dimensional-usually takes form of simulation

Online/eLearning

Another form of technology that is prevalent in today's learning environment is online training or eLearning, which is the delivery of learning and training through digital resources [5]. eLearning arose after the more static CBT training was developed, and is a more flexible and personalized approach to learning that allows the learner to explore and learn based on their own learning preferences and interests [4]. Table 10.2 presents different types of online and eLearning formats.

Both computer-based and online training can be easy to use and provide good opportunities for learners to absorb and practice new skills while making training more enjoyable. They both offer flexible options to allow learners to proceed at their own pace. In addition, both learning delivery options can be cost effective and easy to update with new content. CBT can provide training to many people using the same equipment while online learning can save on travel expenses. At the same time, these options have disadvantages as well. They both require computer literacy by the learners and access to up-to-date hardware. In addition, the learners are required by both formats to work with a certain degree of self-direction.

In addition to CBT training and eLearning, organizations may choose to utilize a blended learning approach which is based on using more than one modality such as instructor-led sessions combined with online learning. A *flipped classroom* approach is an example of blended learning. In a flipped classroom scenario, the learner completes part of the training such as reading content or viewing an online video prior to class. Once in the classroom setting, the learners work together on practice exercises or live problem solving as a group. Using a flipped classroom approach requires knowledge of easily accessible learning technologies that are intuitive and engaging. There are a variety of technologies that are available to provide innovative ways of learning. These learning technologies encompass a variety of multimedia characteristics that appeal to learners. Listed in Table 10.3 are different options that can be used with online learning.

Table 10.2 Online and eLearning formats

Format	Description
Web-based	• CBT modules on the web-available to learners through organization's intranet
Tele- or videoconferencing	• Participants can be in different locations and networked (using the web) into central location-can ask questions of trainer through phone or webchat feature
Audioconferencing	• Similar to video conferencing but involves audio only
Web meetings/webinars	• Dial-in to receive audio training and follow along on computer screens
Online universities	• Known as distance learning-degree programs
Collaborative document preparation	• Share documents through same network
E-mail	• Email can be used to enhance training-follow-up questions and evaluations

Table 10.3 Online learning delivery options

Name	Description
YouTube	• Online video and social media platformed owned by Google • Contains a variety of different videos covering different learning topics
SnagIt	• Screen capture software that captures video display and audio output; customize an image capture and share to favorite program or application-great for software how-to training materials
Video in PowerPoint	• Create videos using PowerPoint
ScreencastOmatic	• Screen casting and video editing software tool used for making videos in flipped classroom situation
Powtoons	• Visual communication platform-can create engaging video with professional look
Screencastify	• Can record, edit, and share videos of computer screen
Panopto	• Screen captures system that allows users to capture audio, video, and entire screens
Flipped classroom	• An example of blended learning that incorporates live classroom learning with online learning
MicroLearning	• Short bursts or pieces of content ex: Videos, eLearning, job aids, games, blogs, podcasts, and visuals

Developing Training Materials

Instructor Guide Examples

After reviewing all the technology options for delivering training, it may be determined that in-person training is still the most effective option based on audience and content. In light of the recent COVID pandemic, another scenario that has been frequently used modifies the classroom training approach, so that in-person training is delivered through a virtual platform using an internet-based communication application as the delivery method. Many organizations, especially health care organizations, are conducting more remote or virtual training as they strive to limit in-person gatherings.

When creating instructor led training, it is important to create a facilitator guide that will provide a comprehensive overview of the different components of the course. The instructor guide creates a step-by-step set of instructions and text for the facilitator. The instructor guide helps keep the instructor on track, providing the right content in the right order so that nothing is missed, and providing delivery consistency between multiple instructors. Instructor guides also contain callouts for emphasizing certain critical content as well as questions and answers to use periodically to check learner understanding. At the same time, learners may also have manuals or guides to use to follow along with the instructor. Learners can use theses guides to take notes, complete exercises, or highlight key pieces of information. An example of an instructor guide is provided as part of this book's resource section.

Learner Manuals, Guides, or Workbooks

As mentioned previously, it is important that learners have a guide to use so that they can follow along with an instructor whether in a face-to face class setting or participating in a virtual session. Often, the learner manuals will be similar in content to the instructor manual. While there are advantages and disadvantages to using paper, manuals can be a very helpful tool for learners to keep them engaged. Having a central online repository or website where learners can go to access the most updated training materials and information is also key. The disadvantage of paper is that information changes rapidly and it is difficult to keep up with paper copies. If learners know where to access the most current information, the chance of learners not knowing the most current procedures decreases.

When learning to use health information technology, learners need the ability to practice what they have learned after the class is over. Developing muscle memory helps learners remember the necessary steps to perform a task within the EHR. Having workbooks with specific exercises included that can be performed in a training environment or *sandbox* will help reinforce important information learned and allow learners to practice remaining proficient, and retain what was learned.

When training multiple learners on a particular workflow within the EHR, it is not always possible to cover all the secondary department specific workflows that each learner will need. An example of this would be training a class of surgeons on how to use an EHR's surgery tools. While the basic function in the EHR for surgeons many be the same, there could be additional tasks, tools and workflows that are needed per each specialty that cannot always be covered in a class setting containing learners from different specialties. Covering each of those specialties is not feasible and creates learner dissatisfaction. Instead, the learners are shown the general workflow and how to perform the main functionality. After class, the learners can use their specific specialty workbooks to complete practice exercises that highlight the different procedures based on their specialty. The general and specific workflow training approach can be a very effective method for training multiple specialties on core EHR functionality and competency.

Testing and Evaluating

Testing

As the training content development nears completion, a testing and evaluating phase can solicit feedback from stakeholders and help ensure that the course contents meet all the requirements and established learning objectives. These stakeholders should be comprised of learners, customers, subject matter experts (SMEs) and other key personnel who are invested in the success of the learning event. Testing the contents during development is highly recommended. To ensure that evaluation of the materials does not interfere with the development of the content, it is recommended that the content be divided into modules so that once a module is completed, it can be passed on to the stakeholder group for review. Finally, performing a thorough review to evaluate punctuation, grammar and ease of understanding is an essential quality assurance step in the process before giving it a test run.

The test run phase allows a sampling of learners to review the contents of the course either through a guided review or through a facilitated learning session where the contents are covered. This test run will provide the learners an opportunity to review the content and provide feedback and suggestions for improvement. It is important to consider the timing or length of the course as well as whether the content and materials meet the needs of the learners. After this step, the finished and updated content should be submitted to organizational leaders for final executive stakeholder approval and to ensure that everyone is aligned and in agreement that the course is ready for implementation. If the training is also going to be performed in-person, a *Train-the Trainer* (TTT or T3) event will be needed to ensure that all the facilitators are comfortable with the materials and processes.

Event Details and Communication

Another important element of developing a successful training event is to plan out the communication strategy, and Chap. 4 provides an in-depth exploration of change and effective communication. This step should start with the leaders of the targeted groups to be trained. The leaders will be responsible for ensuring that their learners are enrolled and attend the training session. This means that identified leaders should meet with the training professional to understand the details of why this training is taking place, and what the process will be for training their teams. Ideally, there should be plenty of lead time provided to ensure that the leaders can work out staff coverage schedules. Leaders will need to plan for ample time to schedule all the members of their teams to either attend a live event or have them go to a designated quiet area so that they may work on the online learning module.

Gaining an understanding of other projects that may be in implementation within the organization will assist the training professional in selecting a timeframe that works best and allows for the least number of competing priorities for the learners. As part of the training plan, consideration should be given to the scheduling method and the process for notification of training. Having conversations ahead of time to ensure that the correct leader contacts are in place will ensure that the communication process runs smoothly. The communication that goes out should include all details related to the training event, including date, time, duration, how to access the training, prerequisites and why the training is taking place. In addition, there should be a point person designated and listed on the communication that can help with any questions about enrollment or logistics related to the training event.

Conclusion

The development phase of the ADDIE model is a true test of how well the analysis and design phases were performed. If there was due diligence performed in the earlier two phases, the development phase should be straightforward and relatively streamlined. The development phase is all about putting everything together to create a fully functional learning experience. Another important aspect of this phase is remaining patient even when the goal is in sight, and ensuring that leaders and other stakeholders are onboard with the training that is created.

Technology has improved the way the world learns, and with those advances, the ways that organizations can train their workforces. By utilizing technology in exciting and innovative ways, mundane training can become engaging, customized, and delivered to users faster than ever before. Training is constantly changing and improving, thanks to the use of creative solutions. By adapting training to reflect current trends, courses become more beneficial to the learners and of greater value to an organization. It is possible to build trainings that are on the cutting edge, designed with the learner in mind, and easily accessible for employees [6]. Finding the right balance between training and technology helps training professionals deliver the best possible courses by the most accessible means, which leads to greater learner engagement and better organizational outcomes.

Discussion Questions and Answers
1. What are the major steps involved in the development phase?

    There are three major steps involved in the Development phase: drafting and prototyping, producing materials, and testing and evaluating. The drafting and prototyping phase is all about building out the learning materials to reflect the design plan. This step involves putting the pieces of content together to produce a draft or *prototype* of the finished product. The next phase on the development journey is to produce materials such as the content, lesson plans, exercises, and potentially eLearning materials needed for the learning event. As the training content development nears completion, a testing and evaluating phase can solicit feedback from stakeholders and help ensure that the course contents meet all the requirements and established learning objectives.
2. Why is it important to evaluate learner profiles when determining the right technology?

    When evaluating learner profiles, the training process is shifting from training at a single location to an increase in remote learning as organizations become less centralized. Many employees are now telecommuting because of the recent COVID pandemic. Since in-person learning may not be feasible, it is important to provide alternative options for continuous learning so that learners are able to stay updated on changing regulations or compliance related items. The ability to train in several locations at once without losing anything in translation is the new reality of health care, and many other industries.

3. Why is it important to test the content developed prior to rolling it out?

   The test run phase allows a sampling of learners to review the contents of the course either through a guided review or through a facilitated learning session where the contents are covered. This test run will provide the learners an opportunity to review the content and provide feedback and suggestions for improvement. It is important to consider the timing or length of the course as well as whether the content and materials meet the needs of the learners.

4. There are a variety of technologies available that can provide different levels of interaction. Discuss some options that you think would help learners stay engaged.

   – Computer-based training (CBT) is a great option that allows for organizations and employees to have more control over the learning process. CBT involves the use of a personal or networked computer for the delivery of training or access to training. CBT can be synchronous or asynchronous, and it can be presented as online, web-based, mobile, and distance learning.

   – Another form of technology that is prevalent in today's learning environment is online training or eLearning, which is the delivery of learning and training through digital resources [5]. eLearning arose after the more static CBT training was developed, and is a more flexible and personalized approach to learning that allows the learner to explore and learn based on their own learning preferences and interests

   – In addition to CBT training and eLearning, organizations may choose to utilize a blended learning approach which is based on using more than one modality such as instructor-led sessions combined with online learning. A *Flipped Classroom* approach is an example of blended learning. In a flipped classroom scenario, the learner completes part of the training such as reading content or viewing an online video prior to class.

References

1. Deick W. Developing real change through learning. Brilliant Learning Systems. LinkedIn; 2020. Retrieved November 27, 2021 from http://brilliantlearningsystems.com/.
2. Treser M. Getting to know ADDIE: Part 3- Development' *Getting to know ADDIE, eLearning Industry*; 2015. Retrieved November 27, 2021 from https://elearningindustry.com/getting-to-know-addie-development.
3. Selecting Educational Technologies: A Checklist. UNT Teaching Commons. University of North Texas. 2022; January 6 Available at: https://teachingcommons.unt.edu/teaching-essentials/teaching-technology/selecting-educational-technologies-checklist.
4. Stoyanov S, Ganchev I, Popchev I, O'Droma M. From CBT to e-learning. J Inform Technol Control. 2005;3(4):2–10.
5. Lawless, C. What is eLearning? Learn Upon Blog; 2018. Retrieved November 27, 2021 from https://www.learnupon.com/blog/what-is-elearning/.

6. Kelso S. Enhancing training through the right use of technology. Educ Technol eLearning Ind. 2019; Retrieved November 27, 2021 from https://elearningindustry.com/enhancing-training-right-use-technology

Kathleen Mandato is the Director of Epic Training & Delivery and the Administrative/Nursing Fellowship Program at Vanderbilt University Medical Center. She has worked in the field of training and organizational development for the last 27 years; 10 years in telecommunications, and seventeen years in the healthcare industry. Kathleen has an MBA and a PhD in Education with a specialization in Training & Performance Improvement. She is a registered corporate coach and is Epic Software certified in the Cadence application. Kathleen also teaches healthcare related undergraduate/graduate classes as an Adjunct Professor at Trevecca Nazarene and Cumberland Universities.

Chapter 11
Training Delivery

Dirk Essary

Abstract This chapter addresses some basic concepts of training professionals and explains practical techniques to improve the effectiveness of delivery. A brief discussion of how to keep training relevant and impactful follow. Finally, a review of how to enhance the learning experience is explored.

Keywords Delivery effectiveness · ADDIE · Methods · Managing distractions

Learning Objectives
1. Understand concepts of training
2. Explain techniques to improve effectiveness of delivery
3. Demonstrate techniques to deliver relevant and impactful training
4. Verbalize actions to take to enhance the learning experience

D. Essary (✉)
Department of Hearing and Speech Sciences, Vanderbilt University Medical Center, Nashville, TN, USA

© The Author(s), under exclusive license to Springer Nature Switzerland AG 2022
B. Kulhanek, K. Mandato (eds.), *Healthcare Technology Training*, Health Informatics, https://doi.org/10.1007/978-3-031-10322-3_11

Training Is Not for the Faint of Heart!

Training is not for the faint of heart—trust me. Several years ago, I was asked to present to a large group of business professionals. Picture if you will a large conference center ballroom set up with round tables for the attendees to sit together and network. The topic had been prepared and the presentation ready to go. The big jumbo screens were glowing and the sound system checked and live. I began the presentation with my prepared introduction and got my audience to respond. The first point went very well and everyone seemed engaged. I checked out my audience of 300 attendees and got into the talk with a little stage flare. It was one of those times when all the elements worked together and you know you are in a groove. As I started to make my second point a gentleman sitting at a table near the stage became a little rowdy and attempted to heckle me. I did what I knew was best and simply ignored him. A few moments later, he graciously repeated his attempt to get my attention. His table mates tried to quiet him and one of them even tried to get him to leave as they knew he had started the evening cocktails early. Another 5 min went by and I thought, all good! Nope! This time he tried to stand as he hurled another verbal jab in my direction. I instinctively knew that I must gain control of the situation. There were 300 other people in this room that had spent their time and money to attend this conference and I was obligated to do my best. I paused, took a deep breath, and walked to the edge of the stage to say, "ladies and gentlemen, I must apologize, I have not recognized a local celebrity, a magician. This man has just tried himself into an ass! Please give him a round of applause!" Well, the man was stunned silent, a table mate directed him out of the ballroom, and the rest of the room applauded his exit. That my friends, is NOT what any trainer should do during a presentation. My point is, even a well-prepared trainer needs to be ready for surprises or unplanned events. Staying in control is key to a successful learning experience. If you are wondering, the session went well but my boss and I had a conversion after the conference about professionalism while training.

Training Skills

Most people do not understand what it takes to truly be a good, effective trainer. Many times, those who inherit or step into this role are not trainers by choice or trade. This fact puts the trainer at a distinct disadvantage as it relates to being successful and more importantly, helping the learner to be successful. To borrow a phrase from Stolovich and Keeps [1], telling ain't training. Whether a trainer has a formal training background or has been selected to share their knowledge because of their demonstrated expertise in an area, there are elements that should be employed to positively impact the learning experience and make the training more effective.

First of all, it is important to consider some fundamental aspects of the learning audience and the environment. The audience consists of those whom the instructor will be leading through the training event. The instructor, or trainer, cannot connect to the audience if they are not aware of the background of the learner, including their familiarity and experience with the topic to be shared, or the formal training the learners may already had on the training topic. If the trainer addresses the group as if they have no knowledge when they are well-informed, the trainer will lose credit-ability and from that point on, the engagement of the audience will decrease. As outlined in Chap. 8, the assessment or analysis step of the ADDIE model provides the information necessary to understand and know your audience.

If training is focused on how to follow an updated version of a process, it can be helpful to engage the audience to understand the current level of knowledge of the issue or process. Querying the audience can provide information such as how many in the audience are seeing this information for the first time. When the level of audience expertise is identified, the trainer is able to emphasize certain points, and only reference new points of information. It is important to remember that no learner appreciates being belittled, therefore the trainer must be sensitive to where the learners currently are during the learning event.

The audience may have concerns that the trainer will need to address, or to direct to another source for additional information. Having a place to note questions and comments not addressed during training, or a *parking lot*, is a good way to keep the learners on track while assuring them that their questions and concerns will be addressed at some point.

The next training delivery point is more technical and relates to the application of learning theory, an important consideration for a trainer. An audience of adult learners is different than an audience of school age children, and adults do not learn the way children do. Children, especially younger learners, learn by simply memorizing and mimicking what their teacher shares. They tend to take most information provided by the teacher as fact and they most often receive and accept information from their teachers. Children as learners do not regularly question the content nor offer options. Children learn according to a manner referred to as *pedagogy*. Pedagogy is the method and practice of teaching, especially as an academic subject or theoretical concept [2]. This approach to learning originates in ancient society and is based on the method of teaching by telling. The science of pedagogy has expanded throughout the centuries but the basic concept remains.

The adult learner is a more complex learner because their brains have gained experience and by adulthood have developed higher functions. There are many scholarly sources exploring the development of the human brain and the reality of the brain's higher function after adolescence. Studies find that the brain's prefrontal cortex, the center of problem solving and decision-making is not fully mature until the age of 25 [3]. The second, and more prevalent fact is that adults need to apply what they are learning to past experiences and to concepts personally relevant to them. As part of accepting training as fact, application is critical to placing value on the information and testing it mentally against previous knowledge and constructs. In other words, adult learners do not blindly accept what they learn. For adult learners, their life experiences must be validated or reconciled as learning takes place.

As the trainer understands how the adult learner processes information and the importance of knowing the demographics of the audience, the next element that impacts the ability to train is the learners' need to maximize their learning experience (Table 11.1). Be aware of learners with physical challenges that may require accommodation such as those with mobility issues, or who are sight or hearing challenged. These basic physical challenges must be addressed before any learning may take place for those learners. In today's workforce, tools are available to assist those with physical and learning challenges and trainers must take full advantage of them, not just for the sake of the learner, but also for those who ultimately receive the actions that are the end product of training. The trainer must never lose focus of the fact that what is being taught is not solely for the benefit of the learner but also for those they help in their jobs. The recipient of care, the patient, benefits from an educated and confident professional. Not only must the trainer consider these challenges, but must also be prepared to address learners with language or cultural differences.

As part of the initial analysis, the trainer must understand if the learners are comfortable with the common language of the workplace. This not only includes terms as part of the health care profession, but also the spoken language. In addition to the language of choice, the trainer must remember that people from various parts of the country or from around the world may use slang phrases with unique meanings with which not all are familiar. It is paramount in training to avoid colloquialisms and only speak using a more formal approach to language. This simple act will assist everyone in understanding the intended training message.

It is obvious that the considerations presented thus far must be evaluated prior to any learning that will take place. The trainer must be prepared to present the training content. Instructors should never treat learning as a casual conversation, preparation and professionalism are important aspects to success in the training role and important for those that are impacted by the learning process.

The final consideration that a trainer must assess and prepare for is the efficient use of allocated time and other limited resources. The classic *ideal* training event

Table 11.1 Training skills and preparation

Skill	Preparation
Know the Learner	Review the training analysis to understand the current knowledge of the audience, teach to the level of the audience
Follow Adult Learning Principles	Avoid lecturing and involve the learner in the learning process. Connect new information to past experiences and concepts familiar to the learner
Consider Accommodations	Ensure that the environment and technology is sufficient to meet the needs of any learners that need adaptive technology or aids
Control Language	Avoid using slang or colloquialisms when speaking to avoid confusing the learners with unfamiliar terms or language
Professional Approach and Appearance	Remain professional in both attitude and appearance so that training is not perceived as a casual event. Professionalism increases the importance to the audience of the content being delivered

versus the pressures of *production* is a conflict that requires balancing the time of the employee away from their job with the benefits of learning. This reality must be addressed by those developing and designing the training and agreement from those managing the actual job responsibilities and staffing for the end user. For example, if employees need to know how to fill an order using a new computer program, the designer determines through development and testing that the average time to understand or gain proficiency of this function is 2 h. In contrast, the manager of the work group can only accommodate a span of 1 h for the employee to be away from their daily function. The classic conflict is that of scarce resources including demand on time and work need. Speaking in terms of economics, it is the concept of basic supply and demand.

Leaders and those engaged in both training and operations functions must collaborate to design a solution that meets the needs of both groups of stakeholders in the real world. Often the solution to the resource conflict is a compromise of resources that impacts both work flow and learning and is unfortunately the reality of learning on-the-job today. The Association of Talent and Development (ATD) defines on-the-job training (OJT) as *any activity that helps employees acquire new, or improve existing, knowledge or skills*, and compromise may involve on the job training (OJT) rather than formal training, or a combination of the two. Training is a formal process by which learning professionals help individuals improve their performance at work. Development is the acquisition of knowledge, skill, or attitude that prepares people for new directions or responsibilities [4].

Once the training delivery solution is determined and the agreed upon training course time and related logistics are set, the trainer needs to continue as they work to manage the information presented in the time allotted. Simply put, the trainer must provide the best content possible in the time allowed for the course. Efficiency in delivery and learning are key skills and the trainer must be careful to plan the learning experience and honor the allotted time and use of resources. It is important to note that the trainer must not comment to the learners about any training challenges, but rather focus on the information to be shared and make the learning experience the best it can be for the learner.

Delivery Methods

There are many forms of delivery methods available to trainers today depending on the resources within their organization. However, this chapter will focus primarily on four delivery methods and their respective options. The four most common training delivery methods are instructor-led training (ILT), virtual instructor-led training (VILT), online learning, also known as self-paced or e-learning, and blended learning.

Instructor-Led training (ILT) is the classic in-person classroom style training. The trainer and the learners are in the same physical location while learning. Most are familiar with this from being a student in primary and secondary education, in college and university settings, and in seminar environments. The advantage of this traditional learning environment is the face-to-face interaction that occurs between all present. The trainer has the added ability to read body language or gauge facial expressions that communicate a learner's understanding or agreement in a non-verbal way. A well-known theory on non-verbal communication is known as the 7–38–55 rule and is a description of how people communicate their emotions. The rule states that 7% of meaning is communicated through spoken word, 38% through tone of voice, and 55% through body language. It was developed by psychology professor Albert Mehrabian at the University of California, Los Angeles, who proposed this concept [5]. Body language also enhances the networking ability between learners to apply new concepts and analyze information so that learning is reinforced. The in-person interaction found in ILT is a distinct benefit not found in other training delivery methods.

Virtual Instructor-Led Training (VILT) is the next delivery option. This method adds a new way of being present by having the instructor and learners all attending through a virtual classroom. Although no learners are in the same physical space, the learning environment is still a collaborative environment. Learners are able to interact with, and see each other. The virtual learning technology used for this type of learning setting is well established in many organizations.

Facilitating a learning experience while the learners are physically separate results in an interaction that is slightly more formal and can create a barrier to learning if the attendees are not comfortable with the program used for the session. The added requirement of using technical skills detracts somewhat from the pure learning element and must be considered.

A distinct advantage to this type of learning delivery is a reduction in the time and cost associated with the travel to the learning site. The savings are more evident when a larger group of learners are coming together from many locations. As our world of learning evolves with technology and changing work options, virtual formats are becoming the standard for many learning experiences.

One particular form of learning that has become an option for learning is known as online learning. Other terms associated with this include self-paced learning, or e-learning. This type of learning adds an extra dimension to the online experience. The word online means simply to be connected to a computer or a computer network. The more descriptive terms of self-paced learning or eLearning provide a better understanding of this concept. Self-paced learning is learning that takes place as a single user participates in an automated course designed to provide interaction between the program and the user. The primary goal is to impart knowledge of a subject. The key difference with this option is that the learner progresses through the program at their own pace. The learner is able to stop and review a section, or repeat a portion of the learning. The learner has an element of control that aids the learning experience.

E-learning adds additional elements to self-paced learning. eLearning offers learning tools within the program such as videos, tests, recorded lectures, learning games, and branching learning. There are several benefits to e-learning versus classroom training including the ability to engage in learning almost any place where you have an internet connection, learning can be conducted at the convenience of the learner, it can be tracked, and it can be far less expensive. eLearning is also scalable to large groups and can be made available to groups that are geographically dispersed around the globe [6].

In many cases the training delivery method is determined by those who design or develop the training. All of the delivery methods have advantages and disadvantages for the learner. The key factor is to determine the most effective and efficient method for the organization's learning goals. These methods may allow for training options that include microlearning, simulations, on-demand training modules on various topics just to name a few. Microlearning is learning that presents a key concept in a very short amount of time with short-term learning activities. The term is used in e-learning to quickly update learners within their working environments.

The trainer's job is to be comfortable with the method and to be prepared to use it for the learner's success.

When training for either VILT or ITL to be successful, the trainer must be able to control the learning experience. The first tool of the trade is engagement. No matter the topic or learning technique employed, if the learner is not engaged all effort is for naught. The learner must be engaged, and they must value the training to actually understand the benefit of the learning experience. Adult learners do not appreciate teaching through lecture, and the adult learner needs to be able to identify what is beneficial in the training for them. The *what's in it for me* question is commonly referred to as the acronym WIIFM. Here is where the adult theory of learning becomes the reality of adult learning. The learner must understand what they will gain from this training. Once that is answered, the next part of the engagement element is keeping the learner involved in the topic.

In situations where a trainer is working with a classroom or a small group of employees, there are environmental factors that should be considered. The first is dealing with distractions. Today's jobs demand that employees handle multiple tasks almost simultaneously and the trainer must contend with learners who are thinking about their primary job while in a learning session. Some implicit distractions are outside of the trainer's control, but others are not. The trainer must control the noise in the learning session as much as possible. If the training is being conducted in a room without doors, it is important to find the quietest area possible to limit workplace noise.

Another simple technique to decrease distractions in a shared space is to position the trainer so that there is only a wall behind the trainer with no other movement visible. Movement not related to the learning content will divert attention to unnecessary or unwanted actions. Cell phones can pose another distracting challenge. Once the learner is committed to the learning session, they must be just as committed to focus on the trainer and not focus on their personal cellphone. A good training practice is to address cell phones at the beginning of the training session and ask that all phones be placed on silent and put away in pockets or backpacks. Training has been designed and facilitated by leaders as a designated time for learning and it is important to not allow others, or technology, to take away time from the learning event. Mitigating distractions is not always easy and instructors must stay diligent throughout each session and be able to adapt if needed (Table 11.2).

Table 11.2 Techniques for managing distractions

Distraction	Mitigation strategy
Noise	Close doors, limit workplace noise, eliminate movement behind and around the instructor
Technology	Request learners to silence cell phones and put them away during class, ensure that other technology such as laptops are closed and stored during class
Focus	Maintain and assess focus by asking questions periodically during the class to confirm understanding or stimulate thinking
Engagement	Use case studies or scenarios to employ a teach-back process
Time	Conduct pre-training timing with the instructor guide to determine approximate length and time for each section of content, follow the instructor guide and avoid being side-tracked by topics not part of the training plan
Questions and concerns	Create a parking lot where questions and concerns that are not addressed during the training can be noted. Follow up after the class and provide responses to the learners

During each training session, keeping learners focused is critical to their success. One way to do this is by asking questions intended to review what has been covered in training. The goal of asking questions is to allow the learners to repeat back and confirm they are hearing the content correctly. The instructor should carefully assess for understanding and if the learners offer something slightly different from the best answer, be ready to share why their response is good and re-emphasize any missing information. Questions can require a simple repeat or confirmation of a fact or more. Questions that require the learner to apply the facts to a situation become case studies or scenarios in action. This is where the adult learner applies their experience as well as the new knowledge gained from the session. In essence, with case studies or scenarios, the instructor is employing a *teach-back* technique. The term may or may not be familiar, but most have used this technique before in work or home life. If a learner can explain a concept back to the trainer and provide an example of how or why it is correct, they are teaching. The trainer has shared the knowledge and when the learner has applied it correctly the training has been successful because the trainer is successful when the student is correct. If the trainer can engage multiple learners to share in the teach back, they will learn from each other as much as from the instructor. The job of the trainer during teach-back is to ensure that learners are sharing accurate information, and the trainer may need to provide additional information as needed.

A variation of the teach back is sharing a question with others. A learner asks a question, and instead of immediately providing the answer, the trainer will allow other learners the opportunity to answer. This again is engaging learners, encouraging knowledge sharing, and building learning. During this process or any part of the learning experience it is important to be focused on the learning objective. The trainer must stay on track and not allow the learners to divert from the subject to other topics. Remember, the trainer is tasked with sharing information on a specific topic or area of concern. Staying on track is a key element for successful learning. It allows the instruction to be clear and eliminate any confusing delivery while also complying with the preset time limit of the session. Maintaining a time commitment is a positive way to keep a good relationship between the learning and operations groups.

An effective way to handling secondary topics that should not be part of the session but deserve an answer is a *parking lot*. This simple technique can save time and provide a means to follow-up with the learners. Use self-adhesive note pads, a large wall board, a dry erase board, or even a designated scribe to track the questions that are outside the scope of the training topic but should be answered. As the session progresses a short list may be created that the learners can see. This parking lot reinforces that the learners are being heard, while allowing the instructor to remain on topic and engaged in their learning. The best practice is for the list of questions from the parking lot to be taken from the session so that training professionals or leaders can develop answers to the questions and distribute them out to the learners as follow-up within a few days after the session. This process not only provides answers to questions and concerns, but also can reinforce learning and enhance the trust of the learning audience.

While the training tips provided have focused on ILT, the same processes can be applied to virtual sessions as well. The common online platforms available today provide for similar interaction. Although the technique may vary from its stated format in the text, engagement is still a necessary reality. One example of a virtual instructor-led engagement focusing technique is to ask a question with a proposed answer or to make a statement and ask by a show of hands how many attendees agree. The point is to keep the communication between learner and trainer open and well-travelled.

Learning for adults is best presented as a collaborative experience. A final note on learning engagement is that the more ways the learner can process the information the more the learner will retain. If the information can be heard, demonstrated, and practiced, the learning is reinforced three ways. The techniques shared in this text utilize the various ways adults learn and process information, resulting in effective learning. More information about learning and the human brain is presented in Chap. 5.

The content of this chapter has been focused on the practical, real-world of training delivery within the work environment. Many dissenters would say that training is a waste of time that takes away from productivity on the job. In fact, the opposite is true, if programs are designed well, they enhance the employee's abilities and job skills. Additional benefits of training are the impact to company loyalty, job satisfaction, and improved morale. One particular study of 337 nurses noted that one positive outcome of training was increased job satisfaction [7]. No discussion of training delivery is complete without exploring common training mistakes and how to avoid or mitigate them.

Trainer Skills

Although it may be difficult to admit, trainers make mistakes. The key is knowing how to acknowledge an issue and effectively move beyond it to stay on track so that learning continues. The list of common training distractors and mishaps include the neurolinguistic slip. A neurolinguistic slip is the unconscious habit of saying um, ah, or other thought words repeatedly while presenting. There are additional trainer actions that can signal to learners that the trainer is not confident of the knowledge, is new to training, is not staying on script or topic, is not managing their time, not focusing on the learners while presenting by having their back to the audience, not anticipating the common questions, and finally, not appreciating the learner's curiosity and thanking them for sharing a point. Initially this list may seem trite, but for the learner, the value of these unaddressed mishaps may have negative impact on learning and multiple occurrences of these items may bring negatives consequences to the learning experience (Table 11.3).

The unintentional use of words while thinking of what to say is a common event for newer or unprepared trainers. When a presenter uses um, ah, like, or another word that is really not part of their message, the repeated word can indicate that the trainer is uncertain, lacks confidence, or is stressed. In reality a neurolinguistic slip is a natural occurrence that happens when attempting to fill a void in thought that is unconsciously verbalized. These slips are behavioral markers that speakers are working hard to find the next word [8]. These slips are not usually noticed by a learner unless the slip happens excessively during a learning experience. For an example, this author observed a trainer using "um" 137 times within a 1-h session. This presentation was filmed and played back to the trainer, who was surprised as they had no idea this behavior occurred. The good news is with practice the trainer corrected this behavior and the neurolinguistic slip was eliminated from their training practice.

Table 11.3 Common training mishaps

Mishap	Strategy and preparation
Neurolinguistic slips	Practice speaking to reduce the tendency to fill voids or thought gaps with um or ah sounds. Most learners do not notice a small number of neurolinguistic slips
Revealing lack of confidence	Present a confidence appearance and attitude to learners, do not share that you are new to training or do not know the materials
Not staying on topic	Follow the instructor guide so that the instruction is linear and delivered as designed
Failure to manage time	Run through a new presentation ahead of time and note the length of each section in the instructor guide, then observe these timing notes when presenting
Loss of focus on the learner	Become familiar with any technology used during training so that there is comfort with the applications. Do not turn away from the learning audience to focus on the technology
Failure to anticipate common questions	Be familiar with the training content and any potential questions that could arise during the class so that questions related to the course can be answered
Resistance to learner curiosity	Use learner questions and curiosity to reinforce the lessons being presented and show respect to the learner audience for their curiosity

The trainer should never share that they are not comfortable with their training assignment. As a presenter or new trainer, the first rule of success is presenting with confidence. It takes times to become more comfortable presenting to a group of people. When the trainer indicates that they are the instructor, but not a good one, the rest of the learning session will be ruined. Just as a patient would not return to a doctor who stated they were not good at their job; the trainer needs to be confident and lead. However, the trainer needs to be honest and share what they need to share while avoiding presenting something that is outside of the scope of the presentation.

Staying within the scope of the session leads to the next mistake to avoid, straying from the training topic. The goal is to present the material designed for the learning experience succinctly and with a clear, direct flow of information. Adding unplanned content or not following the course content may confuse the intended message. The goal of training is not to confuse the learner but to impart information in a clear way. Straying from the learning plan may lead to the next mistake, which is failing to manage the time schedule for the learning event. Staying focused on the proper content helps the trainer stay on schedule. A great way to do this is run through the presentation ahead of time with a clock so that the trainer is aware of how long each part of the session will take to present. The trainer should leave time for questions so that learners are encouraged to participate and apply what they have learned to past experiences. Learner questions are the key to success.

The trainer should be focused on the learners at all times when presenting. If a trainer uses software programs, white boards, or other technology during training, they should not forget that their focus should remain on the learner. In other words, become familiar enough with technology so that attention is not on the technology but on the faces of the learners. The trainer should be positioned during the session to face the learners at all times. Eye contact and facial expressions convey a major part of the learning message and helps learners to relate to the instructor. The instructor should be personable and comfortable with being in front of an audience while using technology.

Finally, the instructor should make every effort to appreciate the curiosity of the learner audience by welcoming questions. Learner questions are part of the process of active learning and are associated with applying what has been learned. Remember to always appreciate the learner's inquisitiveness. When a learner feels comfortable to ask a question and is thanked for curiosity the experience is safer and more positive. An attitude of appreciation encourages the learner to work harder or to continue to evaluate and engage in what has been presented. Engagement and curiosity result in a powerful multiplier of success and application in the real world. Intertwined with appreciation of the learner audience should be respect. Respect of peers, learners, and leaders in the workplace is a critical factor of success for learning and trust. Respect, or lack of respect, can impact the reputation of the trainer as a professional. A trainer who is professional and respectful has a tremendous opportunity to share with others how to improve what they do, helping others achieve their goals while improving the lives of others.

Conclusion

The role and attributes of the trainer are essential to the success of a learning event. A trainer must be able to present in a professional manner, engage the audience, leverage adult learning characteristics to maximize learning, and be able to utilize both an instructor guide and technology to effectively deliver successful training. The trainer works with organizational leaders and the training team to ensure that training is of value to the learning audience and aligns with established training outcomes. Although training mishaps can and do occur, the trainer should be able to minimize both the frequency and impact of mishaps, manage the learning environment, and positively impact organizational outcomes through effective delivery of training.

Discussion Questions and Answers
1. Why is the adult learner a more complex learner than school age children?

   Their physical brain has developed its higher functions as they reached adulthood. There are many scholarly sources supporting the development of the human brain and the reality of the brain's higher functions after adolescence. Studies find that the brain's prefrontal cortex, the center of problem solving, and decision-making is not fully mature until the age of 25.
2. What is the classic conflict between training and operations in a work environment?

   The classic conflict is balancing the time of the employee away from their job for the sake of learning. This reality must be addressed by those developing and designing the training and agreement from those managing the actual job responsibilities and staffing for the end user.
3. What are the major delivery methods/platforms for training?

   The major delivery methods are Instructor-Led (ILT), Virtual Instructor-Led Training (VILT), Online or Self-paced, and Blended.
4. What is the key factor in determining the best delivery method?

   In many cases the delivery method is determined by those who develop the training. All of the delivery methods have advantages and disadvantages for the learner. The key factor is to determine the most effective and efficient method for the organization's learning goals.
5. What is critical for the adult learner in order to gain knowledge from the learning experience?

   The learner must be engaged, and they must value the training to understand the benefit of the learning experience.
6. What is one of the simplest, yet most powerful tools for engagement and learning for an adult?

   Questions—asking questions to check for understanding and helping learners to focus is the most powerful tool.
7. What are the benefits of training for the individual and the organization?

   Training enhances the employee's abilities and job skills, and it positively impacts company loyalty, increases job satisfaction, and boost morale.

8. What is a neurolinguistic slip and how can this be avoided?

    A neurolinguistic slip is a natural occurence that happens when one attempts to fill a void in thought that is unconsciuosly verbalized. Examples include; um, ah, or like. These can be avoided by knowing your content and pacing yourself. Silence is okay for a few seconds. Finally, practice your presentation and anticipate the questions you may get and know the answers.

References

1. Stolovitch HD, Keeps EJ. Telling ain't training. Alexandria: ASTD Press; 2011.
2. Bowling J, Henschke J, editors. The handbook of adult and continuing education. Sterling: Stylus Publishing; 2020.
3. Arain M, Haque M, Johal L, Mathur P, Nel W, Rais A, Sandhu R, Sharma S. Maturation of the adolescent brain. Neuropsychiatr Dis Treat. 2013;9:449.
4. ATD. Training adult learners. 2021. https://www.td.org/education-courses-atd-elements/training-adult-learners. Accessed 27 Nov 2021.
5. Mehrabian A. Silent messages. Belmont: Wadsworth Belmont; 1971.
6. ATD. E-learning: the evolving landscape. 2020. https://www.td.org/research-reports/e--learning-the-evolving-landscape. Accessed 27 Nov 2021.
7. Bartlett KR. The relationship between training and organizational commitment: a study in the health care field. Hum Resour Dev Q. 2001;12(4):335. https://doi.org/10.1002/hrdq.1001.
8. Orena AJ. There's a neurological reason you say 'um' when you think of a word. Massive Science. 2021. https://massivesci.com/articles/speech-disfluency-stutter-learning-brains-neuroscience/. Accessed 27 Nov 2021.

Dirk Essary holds a PhD in Training and Performance Improvement from Capella University and an M.B.A. from Middle Tennessee State University. He has 25 years of experience in training across corporate, government, and academic industries where his roles including training development, training management, performance improvement, and leadership. He is an Adjunct Professor for Union University. He currently is a Senior Customer Relations Manager with Vanderbilt University Medical Center.

Chapter 12
Training Evaluation: A Summative Task or Active Endeavor?

Linda Hainlen

Abstract Evaluation is a key contributor to the success of a training project. Evaluation begins when the initial performance problem is identified and the need for training has been established. Rather than a process completed at the end of training, evaluation is conducted throughout the analysis, design, development, and delivery phases of a training project and continues past the delivery of the training solution. In this chapter, numerous evaluation models are presented along with many tips and tools that support a robust training evaluation process.

Keywords Kirkpatrick model · Phillips ROI · Brinkerhoff's SCM · Evaluation Formative · Summative

Learning Objectives
1. Describe the components of the training evaluation model
2. Identify the difference between formative and summative evaluation
3. Create a learning evaluation plan that includes evaluation techniques for all four levels
4. Utilize a learning evaluation plan throughout implementation to identify and drive success that reaches stakeholder expectations
5. Create an evaluation report to demonstrate whether the plan is on target, needs adjustments, or is meeting stakeholder expectations

Don't Evaluate to Document, Evaluate to Drive Results.

Meeting the Stakeholder's Expectations
The XYZ Healthcare System rolled out a new Electronic Health Record over the past year and the informatics department had been tasked with training

L. Hainlen (✉)
Sedona Learning Solutions, Daytona Beach, FL, USA

B. Kulhanek, K. Mandato (eds.), *Healthcare Technology Training*, Health Informatics, https://doi.org/10.1007/978-3-031-10322-3_12

the nursing staff to use the new program. Sarah, the informatics director, was excited when asked by nursing leadership to give a presentation to report training outcomes at the quarterly leadership meeting.

The informatics team had diligently learned all they could about this great new software program and had created a training class that was informative and engaging. In preparation for the meeting, Sarah went back and pulled the attendance records, the end of class evaluations, and the assessment scores to compile her report. Here is what Sarah was able to report during the presentation:

Sarah's Training Report

- *1,250 nurses were trained*
- *A 15% no-show rate was planned*
  - *A 9% no show rate was realized, so the planning effort provided more than adequate classroom slots and the team was really pleased with the support from nursing leadership in getting people to class*
- *25 nurses from the units had been selected to act as instructors*
  - *5 of them were not able to fulfill the task because of unit or family priorities, but Informatics had planned for this inevitability so they were not caught short*
- *Evaluations were collected from 55% of the students*
  - *The course received an average score of 4 on a 5-point scale*
- *Assessments were administered at the end of the learning event*
  - *92% of students scored 90% or better!*

Sarah enthusiastically presented the data to nursing leadership and was happy to report it was a very successful training effort. She asked if there were any questions as she waited for applause...

After some silence, the chief nursing officer (CNO) remarked that the presentation was very nice, but she had questions. Do the nurses now use the system as trained? Did the training provided contribute to the results targeted by stakeholders?

Sarah responded again with her evaluation data that showed very successful assessment scores were received and overall, the nurses seemed to like the class as the team had put a lot of effort into engaging the nurses in class.

The CNO persisted and asked again if the nurses were using the system as trained and if intended results were being obtained as a direct result of the learning events. Awkwardly, Sarah admitted that her team didn't really know what happened after nurses left the classes. The CNO responded that it was vital to have this information, without it, it would be impossible to determine whether the informatics training contributed to the results.

Evaluation is not something to be done at the end of training as a summative task, but something done throughout the project to identify desired outcomes, drive outcomes, and produce evidence of value added to the organization.

Why Evaluate?

A continuing challenge in today's climate is to demonstrate the effectiveness and overall worth of an informatics training program. It is no longer sufficient to say that a program was effective simply because people liked it or received passing scores on an assessment. Excellence in patient care is the priority for healthcare workers who have ever-increasing demands on their time. Decisions to take time away from patient care must be supported by not only qualitative but quantitative data.

In the XYZ Healthcare System story, Sarah had gathered data to evaluate her program but had missed the mark on what outcomes stakeholders expected; therefore, her data was not of value to them. Often, tasks such as collecting surveys or administering assessments are completed to check the evaluation box without giving much thought to how useful the information is or how the data collected can be used to ensure or drive success. There are even better reasons to evaluate that unlock much more value, evaluation data can be analyzed during program implementation to inform actions that will lead to a desired outcome. At the end of a project, evaluation can then confirm and demonstrate to stakeholders that the outcome has been reached, and that the outcomes resulted from the actions taken based on evaluation.

What does evaluation mean for an informatics training program? Data gathered from evaluation can help an informatics team to

- Improve the training or learning experience
- Keep a project on track by increasing transfer of learning to behavior
- Demonstrate value to the organization through contribution to realized outcome

Evaluating for these purposes may require re-thinking common practices. For example, collecting and analyzing data only at the end of a project is ineffective because it is too late to do anything with the data other than report failure or success. This evaluation is also often approached with fear because the summative task may possibly indicate failure instead of worth. Instead, evaluation should occur throughout a project and should be approached as an active endeavor or tool that provides data about the next steps to take. When used in this fashion, evaluation at the end of a project will only confirm the success that has been tracked and documented along the way.

> Don't be afraid
> of outcomes;
> be afraid of
> not knowing!

Training Evaluation Models

Several training valuation models exist, and a basic understanding of them is helpful when considering how to implement or improve evaluation within your organization. Most are based on the Kirkpatrick Model [1], credited to Dr. Donald L. Kirkpatrick in 1959.

Kirkpatrick Four Levels

In 1959, Don Kirkpatrick, as part of his dissertation at the University of Wisconsin, identified four areas of evaluation that he used to determine the value of a leadership training course he was offering at the time. The four areas are reaction, learning, behavior, and results [2].

1. Reaction—The degree to which participants find the training favorable, engaging, and relevant to their jobs
2. Learning—The degree to which participants acquire the intended knowledge, skills, attitude, confidence, and commitment based on their participation in the training
3. Behavior—The degree to which participants apply what they learned during training when they are back on the job
4. Results—The degree to which targeted outcomes occur as a result of the training and the support and accountability package

Word of Kirkpatrick's work reached the training industry, and his ideas were published in four articles on evaluation in a training journal, and became known as the Kirkpatrick four levels of evaluation. Although the four levels of evaluation became very popular in the training industry, no additional information on how to properly implement the four levels was published at the time. This led to varied interpretations, and most training professionals struggled to evaluate beyond Level 2 learning. Notwithstanding, the Kirkpatrick Model became well established as the industry standard for training evaluation during the 1970s and 1980s and remains the standard even today. The original articles have been republished for ongoing use [3].

In 1994, Kirkpatrick published a book that went into more depth on the four levels of evaluation. Although the learning community had interpreted the evaluation steps as a linear process, Kirkpatrick clarified that designing training according to his model actually begins with Level 4 results. According to Kirkpatrick, trainers must determine the desired results in level 4, and then proceed to level 3 to determine what changes in behavior will be required to accomplish the desired results. Next, in level 2 learning, trainers must explore and determine the attitudes, knowledge, and skill, confidence, and commitment that must be present to stimulate the desired behavior(s). Finally, arriving at level 1, reaction, the task is to present the training program in a way that allows participants to not only learn, but to have a positive reaction to the training program, are engaged during the learning process, and find the training relevant to their work [4].

Philips ROI

In the mid 1970s, Jack Phillips began to develop systematic ways to collect training data and conduct analysis. In examining the data, he wanted to know not only if organizational results were achieved, but if the return on investment was positive. In 1983, Jack published the *Handbook of Training and Evaluation Measurement*

Table 12.1 The Phillips five-level framework

Level	Description
1. Reaction and action plans	Collects information about the reaction of participants to the program, contains implementation plans
2. Learning	Evaluates changes in skills, knowledge, or attitudes
3. Implementation and behavior changes	Explores on-the-job changes in behaviors specific to the training implementation
4. Impact on business	Examines the impact of the program on the business
5. Return on investment	A calculation that summarizes the monetary value of the training results divided by the costs of the training

Methods [5]. He set himself apart from the four levels of the Kirkpatrick model by adding a fifth level, return on investment [3] (Table 12.1).

Jack Phillips' five-level framework became known as the Phillips ROI Model and is typically thought of as an expanded version of the Kirkpatrick model [6].

Phillips' fifth level, return on investment (ROI) , compares the program's overall cost of training to its monetary benefit; that is, whether the monetary benefit of the results is greater than the cost of providing the course. A key component to evaluating at this level is isolating the training benefits and eliminating any non-training factors that may have contributed to the organizational impact. For instance, the training costs can include staff salaries, trainer salaries, materials, food, travel, room rental and other costs. The training benefits could include tangible and intangible benefits such as increased staff satisfaction, decreased patient care errors, decreased staff overtime, and other benefits [7]. The formula used to calculate ROI is:

$$ROI = \left(\text{total program benefits} - \text{total program costs} / \text{total program cost}\right) \times 100\%$$

ROI as applied to training has always been a topic of debate, as it is not easy to isolate the ROI of training in terms of business results. Usually there are other factors that impact business results such as the results of leaders holding staff accountable, departmental process changes, and other unknown factors. In addition, it is difficult to place a monetary value on qualitative results such as increase staff or patient satisfaction.

Healthcare has not fully embraced evaluation of ROI, both because it is very difficult to isolate results in a complex healthcare environment, and because it may take a year or two after project completion to collect the final ROI numbers. However, if the leaders in an organization want to see ROI numbers, the Phillips Model is the gold standard for calculating them [8].

Brinkerhoff Success Case Method

In 2003, Robert Brinkerhoff introduced a new model for evaluation that focused on why a training program worked well or did not work well. Brinkerhoff had found during his research that there are two realities when it comes to learning and

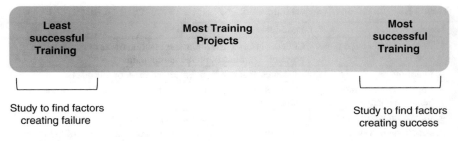

Least successful Training

Most Training Projects

Most successful Training

Study to find factors creating failure

Study to find factors creating success

Fig. 12.1 The Brinkerhoff model

performance that should influence the way we think about and conduct training evaluation.

Training Has a Predictable Impact

In Brinkerhoff's experience evaluating hundreds of training programs, he found a consistent phenomenon; a small percentage of people use what they learn to get great results, and a small percentage of people do not use their learning at all, but the large majority have tried implementing some what they learned (Fig. 12.1). However, these learners noticed little if any positive results and eventually want back to the way they were doing things before [9].

In trying to understand why the impact of training was so predictable, with so few achieving significant positive results, Brinkerhoff found this second reality.

Training Alone Never Works

Like the criticism leveled against ROI evaluation that outcomes can't be attributed to training alone, Brinkerhoff also found that training itself is only one of many factors that influence whether desired training outcomes are met.

According to Brinkerhoff, while it is true that a flawed instructional design, a poor instructor, or poorly designed training materials can keep trainees from reaching objectives, a much larger percentage, up to 80% of failure, is caused by external contextual and performance system factors that were not initially aligned with the intended performance outcomes of the training (Fig. 12.2). Examples include learners not properly prepared to learn, a workplace environment that does not provide opportunities to implement new skills, or a lack of managerial support or incentives for changing behavior. In light of these two realities, Brinkerhoff decided to take a step back and determine if training made a difference for even one person.

Brinkerhoff's hypothesis stated that if he could come up with a credible approach to making the case that training, together with identified performance system factors, had a true impact for one person, he certainly could craft a training evaluation method that could work at the program and organization levels. This formed the foundation for the Success Case Method (SCM) [9].

Preparation & Readiness	**Learning Intervention**	**Application Environment**
• Lack of senior management and commitment • Lack of preparation and focus	• Could not learn it • Wanted to learn, but instruction failed • Facilitator did poor job	• Didn't get manager support • Lack of peer support • No incentive to use • Lack of feedback and coaching

Fig. 12.2   Causes of training failure

The three main components of the SCM include:

1. *Design and conduct a survey* to identify the most and least successful users of the training.
2. *Conduct the success case interviews* to discover stories of success, lack of success, and influencing factors that contributed to or hindered the participants' results.
3. *Formulate conclusions and recommendations* for improving the impact of the training program and for learning initiatives in general within the organization.

The SCM model utilizes the realities of *predictable results* and *training alone never works* to identify factors that contribute to or hinder results to streamline the evaluation process. This model is valuable for improving long-term learning initiatives in which information and findings gleaned from evaluation can help contribute to future learning programs.

New World Kirkpatrick Model

In 2010, Dr. Jim Kirkpatrick and Wendy Kayser Kirkpatrick, seeing that the learning industry was still struggling to implement any type of evaluation effectively, published the New World Kirkpatrick Model (NWKM) (Fig. 12.3). When coupled with the original Kirkpatrick Foundational Principles, the NWKM is a model for planning, executing, and measuring initiatives in a manner that is proactive in ensuring results, not merely documenting results [10].

Based on the belief that evaluation should be an active process throughout a project instead of a summative-only task, the NWKM incorporates elements that connect the dots between the original Kirkpatrick four levels and helps the practitioner make adjustments along the way to ensure that evaluation leads to achieved results.

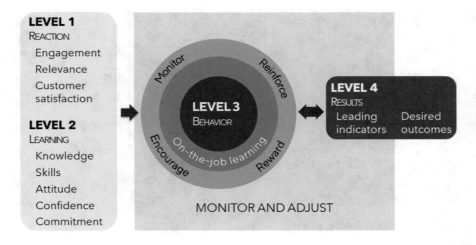

Fig. 12.3 The new world Kirkpatrick model

The key elements of the NWKM within each of the four Kirkpatrick levels include:

Level 1: Reaction—Customer satisfaction with a training program is certainly important, but by ensuring participant engagement and ensuring content relevance, the participant is more likely to learn.

Level 2: Learning—If participants feel confident and committed about using their new knowledge, skills, and attitudes during the learning events, they will be more likely to be successful with behavior change.

Level 3: Behavior—Many factors contribute to outcomes; desired outcomes can only be achieved through partnership. Drivers of behaviors should be identified up front and implemented to ensure results. Required Drivers are processes and systems that monitor, reinforce, encourage, and reward performance of critical behaviors on the job. Examples include checklists, on-the-job learning, encouragement, rewards, etc. If performance is not happening on the job, the model includes monitoring and adjusting to ensure performance.

Level 4: Results—Achieving business outcomes often takes a long time. The NWKM identifies Leading Indicators that performance is on track to produce the desired outcomes. If the leading indicators are not being met, monitoring and adjusting allows for course corrections so that desired outcomes will ultimately be reached.

The added elements emphasize the use of formative and summative evaluation throughout the implementation process so that adjustments can be made to ensure success. This model contrasts with completing and reviewing evaluation at the end of a project to discover whether outcomes were positive or negative and document them.

Table 12.2 Summary of evaluation models

Original Kirkpatrick four levels	Phillips ROI model	Brinkerhoff SCM model	New world Kirkpatrick model
Reaction Learning Behavior Results	• Added a fifth level to the Kirkpatrick four levels which focuses on return on investment (ROI) • Seeks to isolate the monetary outcomes to the training effort alone. Provides a framework for calculating ROI	• Focuses on helping an organization understand why a training program worked well or why it did not work well • Emphasizes identifying factors other than the training itself that contribute to success or failure so findings can be incorporated in continued or future projects	• The model aligns with the organization and proactively drives outcomes so they are not left to chance • Instead of isolating results to the training effort alone, this model focuses on whether the stakeholder expectations are met

Summary of Evaluation Models

There are many models of evaluation. All those discussed here are built on the foundation of the original four levels of evaluation created by Don Kirkpatrick and either add additional evaluation levels to the model, or work to identify success factors for training (Table 12.2).

Operationalizing Training Evaluation

In reality, all the models discussed have value but must be implemented correctly to ensure success. Otherwise, all the effort of evaluation simply documents success or failure. Unfortunately, even after all the attempts to change misconceptions with evaluation, it is still often seen as something that happens at the end of a project in a summative manner only. Perhaps this is due in part to the ADDIE Model of instructional design. The "E" for evaluation comes at the end of ADDIE, which suggests that evaluation is a task to be completed at the end of a project.

However, when training learners to use HIT, training evaluation is understood to be both a formative and a summative task. Training is a planned process that needs to be considered at the beginning of a project, carried out throughout the project, and summarized at the end of the project. It is the process or fluidity of evaluation, not the summative documenting of evaluation, that leads to successful outcomes.

> It is the process or fluidity of evaluation, not the summative documenting of evaluation, that leads to successful outcomes.

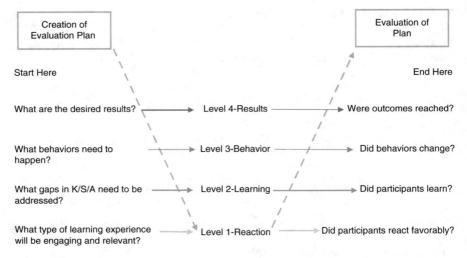

Fig. 12.4 Begin with the end in mind

The process employed by Kirkpatrick, and embraced by other models including Phillips, uses the *begin with the end in mind* approach when it comes to planning evaluation (Fig. 12.4). Understanding the true outcome objectives, or level 4 results, is imperative at the start of a project. This should drive the remaining analysis steps which determine what behaviors are lacking at level 3, and what knowledge/skills/attitudes/confidence/commitment are lacking at level 2.

Although planning begins with level 4 and progresses to level 1, the actual evaluation process begins with levels 1 and 2, and then moves to levels 3 and 4, or level 5 if the desired outcome includes ROI.

The key to creating and delivering a successful informatics evaluation plan is to create the plan at the beginning of the project, in conjunction with the analysis stage of ADDIE, instead of waiting to address evaluation at the end of a project. The plan should then include evaluation within the design, development, and implementation stages.

Project Evaluation Plan Initiation

A full evaluation plan should only be initiated if the project has strategic interest and importance to the organization. Otherwise, the data required by stakeholders and desired by the learning and development team can be identified for other programs and gathered in a less comprehensive and resource-intensive fashion. The Evaluation Plan Determination Form can be utilized to clarify the need to create a project evaluation plan (Fig. 12.5).

Informatics Evaluation Plan Determination Form

Program Name:		Yes	No	Comments
Strategic	Strategic goal alignment?			
	Executive interest/sponsorship?			
	Patient care and/or financial impact?			
Tactical	Managerial reinforcement?			
	Access to training graduates?			
	Is the scope realistic?			
	Is a performance change needed?			
	Is a learning component needed?			
	Is there access to existing level 4 measures?			
	Totals:			

If you answer "no" to one or more of the strategic questions, an evaluation plan may not be needed.
If you answer "yes" to strategic and most tactical questions, consider an evaluation plan.

Fig. 12.5 Evaluation plan determination form

Creating a Training Evaluation Plan

Documenting the problem statement that precipitates a request for training helps define not only the evaluation plan, but the design of the training curriculum as well. The problem statement is typically created during the analysis stage.

Case study application: problem statement
In the last year there has been a 75% increase in catheter-based infections (CBIs) in the intensive care unit (ICU). It is believed that improper technique increases the risk of catheter-based infections. Residents insert the greatest number of central lines in the ICU. The Residency Director hypothesizes that training the residents on a standardized approach to central line insertion will reduce the incidence of CBI. Each ICU CBI cost the healthcare system approximately $82,000 and causes 3 additional hospital days

The main goal of a training evaluation plan is to determine what data would be valuable at each level to monitor and ensure desired results are reached. To ensure success, formative and summative evaluation should be included at each level.

- Formative Evaluation: takes place during the execution of any of the levels while adjustments can be made to ensure success
- Summative Evaluation: takes place after project completion and documents final results

As stated, the creation of a training evaluation plan should take place in conjunction with analysis and begins with level 4 expectations. Following are the expected formative and summative evaluations at each level of training evaluation.

Level 4: What Are the Expected Outcomes?

Summative The first step is to solidify the true expected outcomes from the project. Too often a training request is received and the informaticist goes about creating training without truly understanding the desired outcomes. Most informatics projects align with patient care outcomes, but some projects may be focused on a financial focus and impact. Being able to quantify the expected outcome is important and may need to be negotiated with stakeholders. The expectations need to be measurable and realistic so you know when you have reached the goal(s). For instance, a goal of eliminating catheter-based infections is vague and probably unattainable. Having a good understanding of the problem that exists can help define expected outcomes.

Case study application: expected outcomes
Reduce catheter-based infections (CBI's) in the intensive care unit by 50% for the calendar year

The outcome statement presented is specific, measurable, and obtainable. Most of the time, data at Level 4 is already being gathered by someone at the corporate level or the request would not be generated. For instance, in this example, data is already being collected on catheter-based infections and the data shows an increase in the intensive care unit. These data sources can later be utilized to assess success.

Formative If you implement a training program to reduce catheter-based infections and wait until the end of the year to monitor results, it will be too late to make adjustments. The formative side of level 4 changes the focus from exploring if the training intervention worked, to is the training intervention working. Instead of waiting and leaving the results to chance, identifying the changes that are expected would indicate that training is on target to reach expectations.

By looking for indications that catheter-based infections are decreasing before the year-end reports are available, you can keep your projects on target to be successful. If you are not seeing indications that you are on target to meet expectations, you will want to ensure the right performance adjustments have been made to create the needed change and work with leaders to apply accountability (Table 12.3).

Table 12.3 Level 4 case study application

Case study application—level 4	
If CBIs are on target to be reduced by 50% on the ICU for the year, what might you expect to see? • Fewer infections each month in the critical care unit • Fewer infections for the quarter • Higher patent satisfaction scores from patients who have catheters each quarter • Lower cost of care for patients with catheters	Possible summative reports: • Financial • Risk Management • Clinical Error • EHR System Documentation • Customer Satisfaction (Typically, these are metrics already being gathered that the informaticist can utilize.)

Level 3: What Behavior Changes Will Be Needed?

Summative   Your evaluation plan should include the key behavior changes that will need to occur to reach your desired outcomes that were identified in the analysis stage. It is best to limit the key performance changes to two to four targeted interventions. Behavior changes are actual changes in actions that can be externally observed, not merely theoretical knowledge about how actions are to be performed. For our case study, during the analysis stage it was determined that behavior would need to change in two key areas to reach the desired outcomes of reducing CBIs in the critical care unit:

Case study application: critical behaviors
• Residents perform central line insertions according to validated process
• Nurses demonstrate supportive care according to validated process for patients with a central line

Formative   Change is difficult and typically requires motivation and accountability to achieve. Simply knowing how to do something is not an indication that performance will happen. While building your plan, identify how performance can be driven or encouraged to take place.

Performance is not the responsibility of the informaticist or the trainers. Clinicians, their supervisors, and their managers are responsible for holding clinicians accountable. However, if the informatics training project is to be a success, it will be important to collaborate with and support clinicians, as well as managers and supervisors, so that they have the needed tools, or drivers of performance, they can use to hold their direct reports accountable. These drivers of performance come in several forms, such as reports, reminders, encouragement, rewards, job aids, and so on (Table 12.4). Building a support and accountability package will be key to ensuring success [10].

Table 12.4 Driving performance

Case study application—level 3—driving performance	
How would you monitor and drive performance for the identified behavioral changes? • Residents perform central line insertions according to validated process • Nurses demonstrate supportive care according to validated process for patients with a central line	Possible drivers: • Peer review • Work review checklists and other job aids • Coaching • Observation • Executive modeling • Work review • Recognition • Dashboards • Other_____

Level 2: What gaps in knowledge, skills, attitude, confidence, and commitment need to be bridged?

Summative During analysis, gaps in knowledge, skill, and attitude are determined and learning objectives are formulated. Document learning objectives in the evaluation plan and how learning will be measured. In informatics, some sort of assessment, whether written or performance based, is typically utilized. This assessment should also include measures of confidence and commitment as they are an indicator of performance at Level 3.

Formative Don't wait until the end of the learning events to ensure the learning solution is working. Assess early and often while changes can still be made to ensure success. For instance, a good instructor intuitively assesses during a class to see if participants are engaged and learning, but that information is rarely formally collected to make future improvements to the course. Or, if a particular question is being missed by most students on an assessment, check to see if the instruction was inadequate, or if the learning assessment was worded poorly. Determine if students are feeling confident that they can apply what they are learning. If not, ask determine the reason why the learners are not confident in the application of what they have learned. Often this type of information can be uncovered through conversations and observations. Be sure to identify what information will be helpful at Level 2 and work to build that into the curriculum design and evaluation plan (Table 12.5).

For Level 2 evaluations, begin monitoring with a pilot unit or evaluate the first few classes while changes can still be made.

Table 12.5 Level 2 learning

Case study application—level 2 learning	
How would you monitor and adjust Learning? • Although residents have received training on proper central line insertions, it was determined that a refresher tutorial would be provided followed by supervised practice in the simulation center • Refresher training for nurses on the ICU on proper central line care should also be provided	Possible Level 2 tools and techniques: • Knowledge checks during instruction • Role play • Group activity • Knowledge test pre/post • Presentation/teach back • Performance tests/demonstrations • Instructor feedback • Other_____

Level 1: How will you gauge if participants are reacting favorably to the learning event, and evaluate to ensure that the learners are engaged and finding the content that is relevant to their work?

Summative   The traditional method of Level 1 evaluation is an end-of-learning event survey. However, a survey can be limited and is not always completed or taken seriously. Be sure survey questions are focused on gathering information about the satisfaction of the participant, the content relevancy, and whether information was presented in a manner that supported learning. A variety of options should be considered to get relevant data such as surveys, focus groups, dedicated observers in the classroom, and other methods of data collection.

Formative A formative evaluation explores whether or not the learning participants are reacting favorably to the learning event, are engaged, and feel the content is relevant. If the answers to these questions are not favorable, investigate to identify existing problems (Table 12.6).

Evaluation Dashboard

Once the main outcomes, leading indicators, and measures of the desired changes have been defined, a dashboard can be created for reporting results throughout the project. A dashboard is a tool used to regularly monitor, evaluate, and report the progress of a project for stakeholders.

Defining which indicators to include on a dashboard is often the most difficult step in dashboard design. A lot of data is collected from an active evaluation plan,

Table 12.6 Level 1 reaction

Case study application—level 1 reaction	
How might you evaluate reactions to the learning events being provided?	Possible Level 1 tools • Pulse checks • Dedicated observer • Surveys • Interview • Focus Groups

such as registration for learning events, early indicators gathered from Level 1 and Level 2 evaluation methods that indicate whether adjustments need to be made to curriculum, confirmation that the participants are engaged, and other measures. All this information is useful to the informaticist or learning professional, but may not be of interest to stakeholders. For instance, stakeholders typically expect learning events to be engaging and assessment questions to be clear so reporting small adjustments to these may not be relevant to stakeholders. However, if registration for the learning event is not occurring, it may be important to solicit stakeholders assistance to reemphasize the importance of the training event. If a critical behavior is not occurring, trainers may need to create and apply different drivers or solicit stakeholder participation in holding the leaders accountable for the training compliance of their staff. Choose the top 5–7 data points that will be of interest to stakeholders and show a progression of the project, focusing on Levels 3 and 4 as that information is most pertinent to stakeholders (Fig. 12.6).

By providing regular updates on progress, information can be reviewed and used to inform stakeholders of training progress and insights into any necessary changes to design or implementation. The dashboard should also be visually informative so stakeholders can quickly see if the project is on target and what risks are being escalated and may require stakeholder input or intervention [11].

Having a completed evaluation plan and dashboard provides a roadmap for evaluation that will ensure each project stays on target instead of leaving outcomes to chance (Fig. 12.7). Sharing this plan with the designers who will be creating the curriculum and supporting tools will assist them in designing for outcomes as well as learning.

Training Dashboard As of:

Metric	Target	Actual	Status	Comments/Updates
Registration for Learning	%	%	at risk	
Learning Completion	%	%	behind	
Confidence Score	%	%	on target	
Critical Behavior Progress	%	%	on target	
Critical Behavior Progress	%	%	on target	
Leading Indicator of Success	%	%	on target	
Leading Indicator of Success	%	%	on target	

on Target
Behind
At Risk

Escalation Needed Submit to:
1
2
3

Submitted by:

Fig. 12.6 Evaluation dashboard

Project Name:				
Organizational goal this project supports:				
Leadership sponsor:				
Desired Outcomes				
Problem statement:				
Expected outcomes:				
Outcomes needed by:		Budget needed: Budget approved:		
Other initiatives supporting the project:		Dependencies:		
Critical Behaviors				
Critical behaviors	How will behaviors be supported?	Who will provide needed support?	How will behaviors be evaluated and when? (formative and summative)	What indicators will be realized showing outcomes are on target?
Critical behavior #1:				
Critical behavior #2				
Critical behavior #3				
Learning Objectives				
Learning objectives		How will objectives be assessed and when? (formative and summative)		
Learning objective #1				
Learning objective #2				
Learning objective #3				
Reaction				
How will reaction be evaluated?		What formative & summative evaluation will be gathered?		

Fig. 12.7 Evaluation planning form

Implementing the Evaluation Plan

Once the evaluation plan is created and approved by leaders and the curriculum is designed and developed, it is time to begin evaluation of how the program is progressing during implementation. The initial focus should be formative, evaluating the first phases of the project so that issues can be corrected and performance maximized for the best results during the entire course of the project.

Leaders typically want to see final summative data and informaticists want to ensure positive final outcomes and summaries. This dual need requires gathering formative and early summative data and acting on the data to drive results.

During Learning Events

In the early stages of training events, placing observers in the classroom can help ascertain whether the learning materials are appropriate and of high quality, to assess the receptivity to the instruction, and to view participant responses to the training. The instructor can also provide formative feedback on what is working well and what is not, and this can start with the first classes. Whether utilizing classroom instruction or online tutorials for the learning event, check with early participants or hold focus groups and ask whether the event was engaging and relevant, whether they understood what was expected of them, and what areas, if any, where they struggled.

Gathering early formative and summative Level 1 and Level 2 data and comments provides the information to collaborate with instructional designers to make any needed modifications and ensure the remaining training goes well.

Early Application of Learning/Early Results

Knowing Brinkerhoff's predictable learning impact and the research showing that training alone does not create impact, it is critical that the drivers identified during plan creation are deployed to ensure that changes in behavior happen.

Both quantitative and qualitative information should be gathered early and often to monitor signs that expectations are on target to be met. If indications of success are not evident, informaticists and learning professionals will need to determine if drivers are being applied and if they need to be adjusted to ensure success. As often seen in informatics implementations, one of the first indicators of changing behaviors are complaints that a new system or informatics process is taking more time than before. Taking longer is certainly part of the learning curve when learning new skills; therefore, complaints can be seen as a positive sign that participants are applying what they have learned. Although stakeholders may not be interested in complaints, they will be interested in early comments gathered from participants stating that errors are being caught, or that a new process is working.

Project Title: Executive Summary

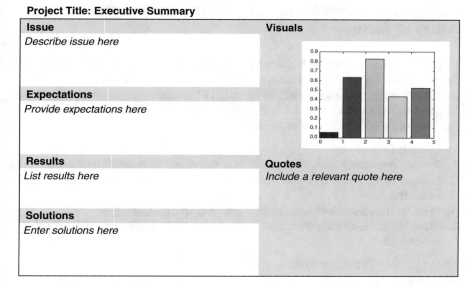

Fig. 12.8 Executive summary

Level 4 Summative Results

If the informaticists or learning professionals have actively worked on an evaluation plan, Level 4 is simply the documentation of final summative results. The good news is that if formative and early summative data has been gathered in time to make adjustments along the way, summative results are very likely to be positive.

Evaluation Plan Reporting

Providing dashboards of progress to stakeholders along the way can be very valuable. Dashboards not only show whether progress towards executive expectations is being made, they provide opportunity for the informaticists and learning professionals to solicit stakeholder support in holding others accountable.

When the evaluation plan is actively monitored and dashboards are created showing progress along the way, a story starts to emerge from the evaluation results. Putting together a final report showing the project evaluation plan and outcomes becomes a simple matter of documentation. A final report not only shows whether expectations have been met, but also documents the plan, the adjustments made, and expected/unexpected outcomes and becomes a historical reference documenting the evaluation project for use with future projects and for documenting the training team's success and performance as well. Keep in mind that stakeholders will likely not be interested in all the details documented. When presenting results to stakeholders, create a one-page Executive Summary, as seen in Fig. 12.8, that tells the story at a glance. Have the full report attached documenting details about the plan for reference.

Summary: Training Evaluation: Summative Task or Active Endeavor?

Evaluation is not a summative action that only takes place at the end of a project for the purpose of documenting success or failure. Evaluation is an active endeavor that is utilized throughout the project to identify if the project is on track, determine whether adjustments need to be made, and to drive results and produce evidence showing value added for your organization.

Discussion Questions
1. In what circumstances would you use formative and summative evaluation?
2. Discuss why training evaluations often contain only level 1 and level 2 evaluations.
3. What techniques would you use to evaluate at all four levels?
4. What are some of the differences between the Kirkpatrick and Phillips evaluation models?

Chip Cookie Evaluation Activity
Your task is to choose a cookie to serve at an event. In your team, define the criteria you will use to evaluate your cookies then score each cookie based on your defined criteria. Each criterion is worth up to 3 points with 3 being the best score. Total the scores to select the cookie you will serve. You will then report your criteria and findings to the larger group.

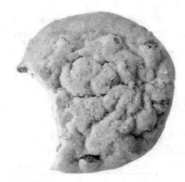

Evaluation Criteria (1–3 points for each criteria) Define Criteria↓ Evaluate →	Cookie A	Cookie B	Cookie C
1.			
2.			
3.			
4.			
5.			
6.			

Suggested Cookie and why_____

_____

_____

Begin with the End in Mind Class Exercise
Before Class

1. Purchase the following:

   (a) Three types of chocolate chip cookies: Homemade, Chips Ahoy, Sugar-free
   (b) Paper Plates
   (c) Napkins
   (d) Sticky Notes & Marker

2. Place one of each type of cookie on plates (about 5–6 students per plate). Label Cookies A, B, C. Cover with a napkin.
3. Make copies of the Cookie Evaluation Form

During Class

1. Place students in groups of 5–6 and provide a plate of cookies and a cookie evaluation form
2. Ask students to come up with criteria to be used to evaluate their cookies. (Common categories students come up with include: chip to cookie, ratio, color, texture, taste, etc.
3. Ask students to score their cookies based on their criteria and come up with a winner.
4. Have students share their results.
5. Now, ask them if their choice would have been different if they had known:

   (a) They were purchasing cookies for a group of preschoolers and the budget is really tight.
   (b) They were purchasing cookies for a diabetic support group

Reinforce the importance of understanding the desired outcome before creating learning materials.

References

1. Kirkpatrick J, Kirkpatrick W. The Kirkpatrick four levels: a fresh look after 50 years 1959–2009. Saint Louis: Kirkpatrick Publishing; 2009.
2. Kirkpatrick JD, Kirkpatrick WK. Kirkpatrick's four levels of training evaluation. Alexandria: Association for Talent Development; 2016.
3. Kirkpatrick JD, Kirkpatrick WK. Kirkpatrick then and now: a strong foundation for the future. Saint Louis: Kirkpatrick Publishing; 2009.
4. Kirkpatrick D, Kirkpatrick J. Evaluating training programs. San Francisco: Berrett-Koehler Publishers; 1994.

5. Phillips JJ. Handbook of training and evaluation methods. Houston: Gulf Publishing Company; 1983.
6. Deller J. The complete Philips ROI model tutorial for beginners. 2019. https://kodosurvey.com/blog/complete-philips-roi-model-tutorial-beginners. Accessed 1 Sept 2021.
7. Herrholtz K. Extend your training evaluation to include the Phillips ROI Model. 2020. https://elearningindustry.com/extend-training-evaluation-include-phillips-roi-model. Accessed 1 Sept 2021.
8. Andriotis N. How to evaluate a training program: the definitive guide to techniques & tools. 2019. https://www.talentlms.com/blog/evaluate-employee-training-program/. Accessed 1 Sept 2021.
9. Brinkerhoff RO. Telling training's story, evaluation made simple, credible, and effective. San Francisco: Berrett-Koehler Publishers; 2006.
10. Kirkpatrick JD, Kayser-Kirkpatrick W. Kirkpatrick's four levels of training evaluation. Alexandria: ATD Press; 2016.
11. Gold J, Riley J, Peersman G. Data dashboard. 2020. https://www.betterevaluation.org/en/evaluation-options/data_dashboard. Accessed 1 Sept 2021.

Linda Hainlen is the Director of Business Development at Sedona Learning Solutions, a Kirkpatrick Certified Facilitator, and an international speaker and author. She served as Director of Learning Solutions for IU Health in Indianapolis, IN for 18 years. Linda has over 25 years of proven experience as a training manager and has worked with companies from around the world to improve their effectiveness and achieve measurable outcomes.

Linda has been published several times, including a white paper co-written with Jim Kirkpatrick on the topic of healthcare. Her ATD Infoline on "Designing Informal Learning" made the top 50 best sellers and was translated into 83 languages.

Chapter 13
Assessing Competency

Brenda Kulhanek

Abstract HIT applications are complex and determining the competency of the end user to be able to safety and effectively use these systems is an important part of ensuring high quality, effective patient care. There are multiple ways to assess the competency of the end user when they use HIT. Although it is not possible to validate competency for each step in an HIT process, it is important to identify key processes where competency can be validated.

Keywords Competency · Behavior · Validate · Assess

Learning Objectives
1. Define competency
2. Explain the importance of measuring competency
3. List two methods used to measure competency

> **Story**
> *The new interdisciplinary clinical documentation system had been implemented for less than a week. To make documentation easier for the nurses, each flowsheet column provided a list of fixed selections to document for each criterion within the flowsheet. At the very bottom of the flowsheet was a small window where additional information could be entered using free text if the information could not be fully captured using the above selections. The nursing staff were having some trouble adjusting to the fixed*

B. Kulhanek (✉)
School of Nursing, Vanderbilt University, Nashville, TN, USA

B. Kulhanek, K. Mandato (eds.), *Healthcare Technology Training*, Health Informatics, https://doi.org/10.1007/978-3-031-10322-3_13

*selection criteria, and one of the nurses started to document all shift infor-
mation in free text at the bottom of the flowsheet column. Within 48 h, almost
every single nurse on that particular unit was using the documentation window rather than the correct processes to document their patient care.
Because the nurses and other providers were not using the correct processes, oncoming shifts and physicians could not see the data that they
needed to make decisions, information could not be seen in graphs to identify trends, and nurses who did not know about the new workaround were
missing data because they did not know to scroll to the bottom of the page!
The organization had to quickly remove the free-text option from the documentation area in the chart to stop the workarounds. Practice drift and
workarounds can happen very quickly and once training has been completed it will be important to regularly assess and provide refresher education about the standard processes that caregivers should be using within
a system.*

Introduction

The ultimate outcome of training is for learners to change their behavior by using
their new skills and knowledge in practice. Changes in behavior and knowledge are
measured through defined competencies. Competency has been defined in multiple
ways (Table 13.1), but regardless of the definition, without competency in practice,
the end result of training is no changes in behavior.

Table 13.1 Definitions of competency

Definition	Source
Behaviorism refers to competency as an ability to perform individual core skills and is evaluated by demonstration of those skills	[1]
Trait theory considers competency as individual traits necessary for effectively performing duties (knowledge, critical thinking skills, etc.)	[1]
Holism views competency as a cluster of elements, including knowledge, skills, attitudes, thinking ability and values that are required in certain contexts	[1]
Nursing competency is generally viewed as a complex integration of knowledge including professional judgment, skills, values and attitude, indicating that holism is widely accepted	[1]
In nursing practice, nurses are required to apply their acquired knowledge, skills and innate individual traits to each situation and be able to adapt that knowledge and those skills to different circumstances	[1]
The ability to perform a task with desirable outcomes under the varied circumstances of the real world	[6]
The effective application of knowledge and skill in the work setting	[7]

Assessing Competency

Identify Primary Competencies

Health information technology applications are typically very complex, and the competencies needed for each learner discipline or specialty will be different than other learners and specialties [2]. It would be impossible to validate competency in every single process found within an HIT application, and there would never be enough time to identify and validate all processes. Therefore, it will be important to identify key processes for each learner group that will be the focus of competency validation. There may be individual processes identified by leaders that will be essential for learners to perform, such as reviewing, acknowledging, and carrying out physician orders, while other competencies may be more general, such as demonstrating the overall ability to admit a new patient to a hospital. It will be important to also consider technologies that interface or interact with the new HIT that is being implemented, such as changes in communication processes or other workflow issues.

Leaders and subject matter experts can provide the insight needed to identify the activities that are key to each role so that competency can be demonstrated. It will also be important to maintain a record of demonstrated competency for each learner for legal defense in case there are subsequent medical errors that are related to patient care and the use of HIT. Additionally, ongoing review of competency should be incorporated into the healthcare organization's routine competency validation plan.

Competencies for utilizing HIT are interwoven with the clinical actions, skills and competencies used for patient care. Both clinical and HIT competency skills utilize three domains of action; (1) clinical/technical skills, (2) critical thinking skills, and (3) interpersonal skills [3]. The use of these three domains in HIT are slightly different than those used for clinical care, but are very interrelated. Examples of this interrelationship include possessing the competency skill of critical thinking seen as the ability to identify the need to assess a certain aspect of a patient, the clinical competency to correctly assess the patient, and then demonstrating the competency of technical skills to locate and document in the correct HIT location. Continuing with this example, interpersonal competency is demonstrated when the nurse communicates with the patient, physician, or other nurses in an appropriate manner and the HIT communication skills may be demonstrated through use of secure texting or the selection of the appropriate methods for communication that are facilitated using technology.

Competency may be demonstrated after training is completed when the learner successfully demonstrates an entire process without error, such as an admission or discharge; or competency can be validated at multiple points in the learning and development process. Additionally, assessment of competency in a classroom setting does not fully provide the real-world environment that learners will encounter as they use their new skills and knowledge in practice. A multi-layered approach to competency validation for HIT skills may provide validation of the basic skills needed to safety begin working, with a second validation of competency after a period of practice.

Table 13.2 Competency validation methods

Competency validation method	Assess during training	Assess in the real-world environment
Tests	Successfully completes a post-test that accurately integrates knowledge into the real-world clinical environment	Successfully completes a post-test that reflects retention of training knowledge and integration of the clinical environment
Return demonstrations	When presented with a process in class, is able to successfully demonstrate the same process	Is able to correctly demonstrate a process during observation (either formal or informal)
Evidence of daily work	Successfully completes an assigned exercise during training	HIT reports and monitors indicate no errors or missing documentation
Mock events	When presented with a real-life scenario, learners are able to demonstrate competency when using HIT to respond to the scenario	When presented with either a real-life event, or a mock event designed for clinical education, learners are able to demonstrate competency when using HIT to respond to the scenario
Quality improvement monitors	During training, instructor reports indicate key processes are completed to fulfill training requirements	Chart audits and reported information that can identify one learner can be used to validate competency, or address competency needs

There are many ways to validate competency, in fact in the clinical care realm there are 11 methods for competency validation according to Wright [3]. The 11 methods for clinical competency validation are (1) tests, (2) return demonstrations, (3) evidence of daily work, (4) case studies, (5) exemplars, (6) peer review, (7) self-assessment, (8) presentations, (9) mock events, (10) quality improvement monitors, and (11) discussion groups. When dealing with HIT competency assessment, some of the 11 methods for demonstrating competency, such as a discussion group, may not be an appropriate method for validating competency. Self-assessment is a method of competency validation that is appropriate only in very specific circumstances such as a reflection of attitudes towards new knowledge and skills. Of the 11 methods of competency validation, five are the most appropriate for validation of learning competency in the HIT learning environment (Table 13.2). Using these methods, validation of competency can be woven into HIT training, or implemented after training so that a record of competency can be maintained.

Align Competencies with Learning Objectives

As training is developed and learning outcomes are defined, the final step in the process is to identify how the learner will demonstrate the acquisition of knowledge and skills in a way that involves application of this new knowledge in a

Table 13.3 Learning outcomes and competency statement

Learning outcome	Competency statement
At the conclusion of training the learner will be able to log into the system	• Learners can demonstrate a successful login to the HIT system when caring for patients
At the conclusion of training the learner will be able to verbalize the reason for patient privacy and security	• Learners can demonstrate proper security procedures when using HIT such as logging off when away from the computer and securing the screen • Learners can discuss the importance of patient privacy and security and how HIT is used to support privacy and security
At the conclusion of training, the learner will be able to navigate within the EHR to locate flowsheets, order entry, and the patient history in the chart	• The learner will be able to navigate within the HIT system to find an I & O flowsheet, enter an order, and locate the patient history
At the conclusion of training the learner will be able to review, acknowledge, and enter an order	• The learner demonstrates the process of reviewing, acknowledging, and entering an order • Based on unit reports, the learner acknowledges all orders within 60 min

real-world environment. Competency assessment can present a challenge as learners in a training environment are not able to demonstrate how they would use their new knowledge and skills in a real-world environment. When learning objectives are established using Bloom's taxonomy, a competency validation is typically the sum total of multiple learning objectives associated with processes (Table 13.3).

Evaluate the Need for Competency Assessment and Documentation

As stated earlier, the number of competencies that could be identified when learning HIT systems would be too numerous to calculate. Therefore, key competencies that are associated with safety, quality, or communication may be identified by a group of collaborative stakeholders to ensure that learners are able to perform safely as a novice system user. There is typically a fine balance between over-validation of competencies when learning to use HIT, and under-assessing competence. When the competence of a new learner is under-assessed, the learner may experience decreased efficiency when using the system, they may feel frustrated, and may commit errors based on a lack of system knowledge and confidence. On the other hand, over-validation of competency can delay highly valued care workers from performing their jobs due to extended training. When this occurs, the organization may baulk at the extra time and cost that it may take to ensure a high level of learner competency, and the learners themselves may be anxious to use their newly learned knowledge and skills while performing patient care.

When post-training competency validation is focused on identified key skills and these skills are measured several times during the training or post-training process, a balance can be maintained between ensuring safe practice through highly competent staff and decreasing safety and quality by under-assessing competency. With the input of key leaders and stakeholders, leaders in the organization will be able to understand and support the training plan and will be confident about the length of training time needed to meet the agreed upon goals.

Identify Methods to Evaluate HIT Training Competency

Although a learner does not lose competency once it has been attained, they can certainly lose proficiency in a skill or task without regular practice or enforcement [3]. When a healthcare provider loses proficiency, it is mostly likely because they have not used a process since they were trained, or rarely use the process. This can occur when a nurse is taught how to document blood administration in training, but when blood is infrequently administered in their daily work, they may lose proficiency and need some reminders for how to complete a certain process. In cases such as this, the learner has not lost their competency, and with the support of readily available quick guides or cheat sheets the learner can review information and quickly demonstrate their initial competency once again.

Workarounds and practice drift are other phenomena seen in HIT [4, 5] which results in unauthorized shortcuts or omissions that can result in errors and incorrect patient data. Ideally, competency should be assessed on a regular basis to ensure that practice drift or shortcuts have not been infused into the routine processes of HIT users. Many organizations will include HIT competencies in the yearly staff competency validation processes so that staff have a built-in opportunity to refresh their memory on correct processes and to demonstrate their current skills. When the key processes are identified and presented as candidates for competency validation, system reports and dashboards can be identified or developed that can quickly show when processes are not being followed within guidelines. Failure to quickly address practice drift or workarounds can create safety issues resulting in errors, can stop the flow of data and communication to all system users, and can skew or impact data that is reported to regulators and used within a system.

Summary

Validation of learner competency is the final step of assessment that demonstrates the learner's ability to apply their new knowledge and skills in a real-world environment. Because a classroom environment is not a real-world environment, competency validation may be best performed using a two-step process. In the first stage key skills identified by collaborating with leaders are validated in the classroom to ensure that novice HIT system users are safe to perform basic functions. In the second stage, competency in advanced HIT skills can be monitored through system reports, dashboards, observation, and by incorporating specific competency assessments into a routine process such as aligning with the yearly nursing skills competency validation process.

The HIT skills competency validation plan should be developed with the inclusion of clinical and organizational leaders because competency validation performed in HIT training can add to the training timeline and increase the cost. With leader involvement, the right balance between safe practice and training efficiency can be managed. Records of competency assessments should be maintained by the training team so that information is available for regulatory review, human resource processes, and for measuring training and the impact of competency validation on organizational performance.

Discussion Questions
1. Describe two methods for assessing learning competency when using the HIT system.
2. Why is assessing competency important? What are the ramifications if learners are not competent?
3. Provide at least two methods for assessing changes in behavior after training to assess competency.
4. Discuss how to address practice drift in an organization.

References

1. Fukada M. Nursing competency: definition, structure and development. Yonago Acta Med. 2018;61(1):001–7. https://doi.org/10.33160/yam.2018.03.001.
2. Voorhees RA. Competency-based learning models: a necessary future. New Dir Inst Res. 2001;2001(110):5–13.
3. Wright D. The ultimate guide to competency assessment in health care. Minneapolis: Creative Health Care Management; 2005.
4. Golay D. An invisible burden: an experience-based approach to nurses' daily work life with healthcare information technology. Uppsala: Uppsala University; 2019.
5. Patterson ES. Workarounds to intended use of health information technology: A narrative review of the human factors engineering literature. Human Factors. 2018;60(3):281–92.
6. Benner P. From Novice to Expert. Am J Nurs. 1982;82:402–7. https://doi.org/10.1097/00000446-198282030-00004.
7. Del Bueno DJ. Experience, education, and nurses' ability to make clinical judgments. Nursing & Health Care. 1990;11(6):290–4.

Brenda Kulhanek is an associate professor at the Vanderbilt University School of Nursing and has a history of leadership in both informatics and clinical education. Dr. Kulhanek holds a PhD from Capella University and a doctor of nursing practice (DNP) from Walden University. She is board certified in nursing informatics, nursing professional development, and executive leadership. Her publications include informatics textbook chapters and multiple informatics articles. She recently participated in the Scope & Standards for Nursing Informatics publication. She teaches informatics at the master's and doctoral levels and has a particular interest in strengthening nursing through nursing informatics education, and the integration of informatics into practice to support improvement of patient outcomes.

Chapter 14
Sustaining Learning

Kathleen Mandato and Dirk Essary

Abstract Despite the best training efforts, HIT processes and procedures may drift from how health care professionals were originally trained. This chapter identifies methods of ongoing learning and training practices that can ensure minimal practice drift. It is also important to maintain and update training content when ongoing HIT changes impacts the learning context. Finally, best practices for managing workarounds are reviewed.

Keywords Continuous learning · Upgrades · Surveys · Workarounds

Learning Outcomes
1. Identify methods to assess ongoing practice and learning
2. List ways to successfully manage the training for software upgrades and other technology changes
3. Discuss best practices to utilize for managing deviations and workarounds

K. Mandato (✉)
Epic Training and Delivery and Administrative/Nursing Fellowship Program, Vanderbilt University Medical Center, Nashville, TN, USA

D. Essary
Department of Hearing and Speech Sciences, Vanderbilt University Medical Center, Nashville, TN, USA

B. Kulhanek, K. Mandato (eds.), *Healthcare Technology Training*, Health Informatics, https://doi.org/10.1007/978-3-031-10322-3_14

Continuous Learning

Continuous learning is an important part of the learning process that requires successful organizational and leadership support. As technology changes, organizations must change to adapt to those changes, and this requires frequent training for the workforce to gain new skills that allow staff to keep up with their rapidly changing roles. A continuous learning organization can remove barriers to HIT assimilation [1]. As noted by Malec [2, para. 12], "The 2021 Global Human Capital Trends Report found that 725 of executives worldwide pinpointed their employees' ability to adapt and learn new skills as a priority for navigating future disruption-and continuous learning is key here."

Continuous learning associated with health information technology can be delivered in a variety of ways. The desire to learn more about developments in one's field or to learn a new skill for an upcoming project are examples of continuous learning. Not only does this benefit the learner, but it also promotes knowledge sharing and increased engagement among staff. To stay abreast of changes within and outside the organization, it is important to evaluate current practices and training programs to ensure relevance and effectiveness.

Deviations or Workarounds

The learning experience is not a single self-contained occurrence that produces the same result for all learners. Dealing with real people in the real world represents an imperfect learning environment with the inherent challenges of retention of facts and behavior modification. Learning requires an individual to retain new information and processing that information may not always be successfully accomplished. As a result, people will deviate from a new process, miss a key step, or overlook an important fact. Poor application of learning is a given, the question is not that it will happen, but how soon it will happen. Sustaining new learning requires innovative ways to stimulate not only learning, but also recall. In the process of learning new procedures, the learner must not only learn new steps, but also to modify what they know of previous processes. Repetition of a new process is a key way to successfully reinforce, remember, and modify behavior.

The Ongoing Training Plan

As part of the training process a plan should be in place to reinforce learning and create periodic evaluations to confirm that new behaviors continue to be demonstrated. For most people, practicing aids the incorporation of new learning into memory. Evaluations may involve observing new learners to view them executing new processes. Direct observation is also a great opportunity to reinforce learning by acknowledging and reinforcing successful practices. During observation there is opportunity to provide any correction or necessary adjustments so the learner is successfully executing each task. It is important to encourage those who may struggle with change and praise the steps done correctly when they handle a task accurately.

Acknowledgement of the successful application of learning is a classic technique used to reinforce accuracy and build confidence. Additionally, following up with a learner helps to assure that everyone is using the same information, processes, and procedures. When all learners are consistently performing the same actions, increased quality and higher reliability is seen in healthcare due to consistency in performing processes. Consistency also facilitates others to handle their tasks more efficiently while increasing the quality of execution.

All learners need to understand why each new process is important. Explanations of change may include why the process changed and the designed benefit to the program, the user, and the patient. Providing explanation of change in the context of the benefit to the patient and the learner is an impactful way to reinforce the *why* in learning. Providing the rationale for change reminds the learner of the strategic benefits of the change, and those changes have an impact much larger than one individual following a particular process. Just as important as sharing the rationale and benefits of the change is sharing the consequences of not learning the new process and how others, including patients, can be impacted. Understanding both positive and negative strategic consequences is a powerful way to motive learners to modify their behavior.

An unfortunate reality of the workplace is that workarounds occur, sometimes unplanned and sometimes for necessity until a technical process is corrected. Developing or using a work-around or alternative path to complete a process or task should not be an individual decision. The alternative path should be documented and tested as a short-term process while the system in question is upgraded or enhanced. Additionally, any alternative processes should always maintain system integrity and validity.

Upgrades

An important part of maintaining technology and continuous learning in an organization is ensuring that there is a process in place for managing software upgrades. A software upgrade refers to any major changes in the system that add significant enhancements or provide new features to the program. Upgrades provide valuable functional and regulatory updates that enhance the overall performance of the system and provide opportunities for additional capabilities that may enhance the learner and patient experiences.

Training is a critical step in the process of implementing upgrades that requires adequate planning and resources. In addition to their regular workload, trainers must carve out time to begin studying the upcoming anticipated changes as well as spend time understanding how those changes impact the system and users. The amount of training and type of training will depend on the feature changes. Most often, training materials such as manuals or tip sheets can provide sufficient guidance to the users to help them prepare for the upcoming changes. Other times, the changes are more in-depth and require classroom training or online training. In any case, upgrades often provide the opportunity for learning that requires lower impact just-in-time training with the least amount of distraction or loss of productivity to ensure a smooth transition.

The first step to developing a training plan for an upgrade is to determine a training strategy that includes multiple modalities that will help users learn the material to the best of their ability. There are various methods to consider based on the complexity of the upgrade. As mentioned previously, in most cases, having a central repository where learners can go to see what the changes are that will impact them is all that is needed. The resources provided can include a manual or tip sheet that outlines the change, a screenshot depiction, or provision of additional information on how to use the new or changed feature. One recommendation is to create guides or manuals by user role that are available on an easily accessible central online site that can be updated as needed. Most software contains functionality that is organized by role. Creating role-based user guides will provide an organized manner for learners to search for changes and associated educational materials that pertain to them.

Another example of training that can be provided in addition to tip sheets and user manuals is microlearning. Microlearning it typically a short burst of information with a specific learning outcome relayed in a variety of formats. A quick video outlining some of the major changes and why they are important can be very helpful for auditory learners, and provides the ability to provide the why behind the changes which will help all learners with commitment and buy in. Learners must understand and accept the reason why they need to make the effort to understand and navigate through the changes. Whether included in the training or contained in the communication strategy, helping to explain the why and the benefits associated with these changes will have lasting effects on how successful the learners will be in completing the training and using the system. A final element that will help support this process and encourage a positive outcome is enlisting the support of leadership. This can be achieved by having them review the training prior to rolling it out to the users to ensure that they understand the changes coming and are in a good position to help their staff.

Evaluation Methods

Surveys to Track Success

One common tool to help trainers understand what the learners are struggling with is a survey. Often, those who design the training will also design a survey as a way to track successes and challenges. Trainers should welcome surveys that are designed to rate content and the success of learning implementation. These surveys can provide the trainer with a keen insight on the specific needs of the learner.

Surveys can be either informal or formal. The informal survey is a quick way for the trainer to understand how the learner is doing and can be accomplished in one of three ways. First, the learning professional can ask questions of the end users. Discussion is a powerful tool and it is important to ask the right questions and listen to the responses from the learner. Because change is often stressful for the end user, personal discussions should display empathy and concern.

When end users are new to using an EHR or other technology, they may not know enough to ask the right questions. Be prepared to restate or paraphrase unclear questions to make sure you understand the nature of the question. Provide an environment where the end user can feel free to ask any questions, and acknowledge that the question is valid while providing an answer. To stimulate the critical thinking of the end user, the learning professional can also ask the end user what they think the correct answer to their question might be. This provides the opportunity to reinforce knowledge or clarify gaps in knowledge.

A second way to survey learners is to send an email or other form of communication that contains one or two questions that are open-ended and allow for feedback. Seeking feedback using an indirect survey method such as this may make learners more comfortable with sharing, and more information may be obtained. It is very important to take the time review survey responses and to follow up. If it is not possible to reply to questions asked in this type of survey, it is best to either avoid this type of communication, or create a Frequently Asked Questions (FAQ) document that all end users can view. A lack of response to the end users after a survey can damages the ability to encourage communication in the future.

A third method for obtaining end user feedback is through the use of a formal survey such as a questionnaire. A questionnaire is more often distributed in an electronic format with a frequently used method for collecting responses. Response options can include rating scales, descriptive responses, or levels of measurement (Table 14.1). After survey responses have been collected, the survey results are analyzed and trends are noted. The formal questionnaire type survey is designed to focus on pre-determined areas. As such, these surveys have limitations and can be perceived as impersonal. To address this, surveys can include open-ended questions or comment boxes that ask for additional details. When properly designed, surveys are proven to be very effective in collecting opinions, viewpoints, and facts. It is important to note that the design of the survey is a major factor in how the survey is perceived by the end users and in the content the survey is able to collect. Notably, formal surveys typically take longer to obtain final results that can be shared with others. Both informal and formal surveys serve a purpose and can offer valuable insight into the learning experience for trainer and learner.

Purpose	Example
Dichotomous Questions	
These types of questions force a decisive response, which removes any opportunity for vague or ambiguous answers. Examples include responses such as yes/no or true/false. However, these types of questions are less reliable due to the likelihood of making a choice of the correct answer through guessing.	○ Yes ○ No ○ True ○ False
Measurement Scales: Ranking	
Provides an opportunity to gauge preferences by allowing selection of fixed items from most to least preferred	**Order the seasons from your most favorite to least favorite.** – Spring – Summer – Fall – Winter
Measurement Scales: Likert	
A Likert scale provides for a comparison of an item along a continuum. This type of scale might have a range from very positive to very negative and allows for one response per subject	**I liked the presentation:** ○ Strongly Disagree ○ Disagree ○ Neutral ○ Agree ○ Strongly Agree
Measurement Scales: Interval	
An interval scale provides a ranking of equally valued responses along a continuum and is used to gauge the spectrum of preferences, likes, and attitudes	**Rate how you enjoyed the presentation.** 1 2 3 4 5 6 7 8 9 10 Worst ──────────────▶ Best
Measurement Scales: Multiple Choice	
A multiple -choice scale provides a wider range of potential responses, while requiring the choice of a specific correct answer. Is often use d to test knowledge.	**What is the color of the sky?** a. Blue b. Red c. Green d. Yellow
Measurement Scales: Multiple Response	
Questions containing a list of pre -selected items which require identification of what items apply or do not apply	**Check the responses that indicate how you felt about the presentation:** ☐ Engaging ☐ Boring ☐ Inspiring

Table 14.1 Survey methods

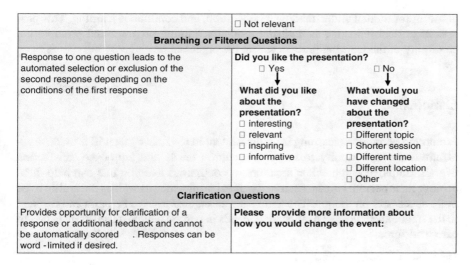

	☐ Not relevant	
Branching or Filtered Questions		
Response to one question leads to the automated selection or exclusion of the second response depending on the conditions of the first response	**Did you like the presentation?** ☐ Yes　　　　　　　☐ No **What did you like about the presentation?** ☐ interesting ☐ relevant ☐ inspiring ☐ informative	**What would you have changed about the presentation?** ☐ Different topic ☐ Shorter session ☐ Different time ☐ Different location ☐ Other
Clarification Questions		
Provides opportunity for clarification of a response or additional feedback and cannot be automatically scored . Responses can be word -limited if desired.	**Please provide more information about how you would change the event:**	

Tab. 14.1 (continued)

Curriculum Review Sessions

Another method that is associated with continuous learning is creating a schedule and carving out a periodic time to review current training curriculum to ensure relevance and that any changes to the curriculum are noted. The main purpose of a periodic curriculum review is to optimize the learning outcomes of the curriculum and improve the overall learner experience. Training professionals should try to stay apprised of updates or operational changes that may impact their curriculum, and make note of these changes for future curriculum updates if the change is not immediate. Sometimes changes are made to the technology or processes without the knowledge of the training team and this can impact the accuracy of the curriculum.

Training professionals should also conduct curriculum review sessions that include a sampling of the targeted learners and their leaders associated with a particular curriculum to verify the accuracy and relevance of the curriculum. Small review sessions can be coordinated with end users and during these sessions the training professional will review the current curriculum section by section to obtain feedback or suggestions. The goal is to identify gaps and ways to improve the learner experience. Once the session has been conducted, the detailed notes are reviewed, shared, and the training professional can make the necessary changes to the curriculum. After updates, the revised curriculum is reviewed a second time with the same audience to obtain approval. After final approval, the curriculum is ready to be implemented. Ensure that the trainers that are delivering the curriculum have sufficient time to review the changes so that they are fully prepared for the next class.

Curriculum review sessions not only highlight the changes needed but they also provide an opportunity to recognize the effectiveness of the curriculum. The partnership established between training and the operations team provides a solid platform for mutual understanding, cooperation, and continuous learning. This process of critical reflection will ensure a quality training program and promote the credibility of the learning process within the organization.

Conclusion

Promoting continuous learning is an investment in the future that will provide organizations the opportunity to improve retention levels and employee satisfaction overall. Employees appreciate a culture of continuous learning that can help them achieve their personal goals, such as technical proficiency as well as the ability to be more successful on the job. The ability for an organization to be agile and respond to the frequent changes in healthcare depends in part on having a well-trained health care workforce.

Discussion Questions and Answers

1. Why is continuous learning important and what does it accomplish?

   Continuous learning promotes knowledge sharing and aids individuals in staying abreast of changes within the organization. This allows evaluation of current practices and training to ensure relevance and effectiveness.

2. What are some best practices to address deviations or workarounds?

   One example of a best practice is to reinforce learning by offering periodic evaluations that help confirm new behaviors are being followed and when they are not being implemented in the workplace. Another example is to conduct a follow-up to check for understanding and reinforcing the reason for change. This method is also a valuable tool, for placing importance on the behavior.

3. What are some of the benefits of conducting a curriculum review session?

   A key benefit of conducting a curriculum review is the ability to highlight needed changes, as well as an opportunity to celebrate the strengths of the curriculum. This ensures program quality and promotes credibility of the learning process.

4. Explain the importance of having a central repository of training materials for an upgrade?

   A centralized repository offers a common, well-defined location that all learners may access. This allows learners easy access to tips, guides, etc. while helping the learner understand the changes and the impact to relevant processes.

References

1. Sánchez-Polo MT, Cegarra-Navarro JG, Cillo V, Wensley A. Overcoming knowledge barriers to health care through continuous learning. J Knowl Manag. 2019;23(3).
2. Malec M. Continuous learning: what it is, why it's important, and how to support it. 2021. https://www.learnerbly.com/articles/continuous-learning-what-it-is-why-its-important-and-

how-to-support-it#:~:text=%20How%20to%20Practise%20Continuous%20Learning%20
with%20Purpose,hasn%E2%80%99t%20hel. Accessed 26 Sept 2021.

Kathleen Mandato   is the Director of Epic Training & Delivery and the Administrative/Nursing Fellowship Program at Vanderbilt University Medical Center. She has worked in the field of training and organizational development for the last 27 years; 10 years in telecommunications, and 17 years in the healthcare industry. Kathleen has an MBA and a PhD in Education with a specialization in Training & Performance Improvement. She is a registered corporate coach and is Epic Software certified in the Cadence application. Kathleen also teaches healthcare related undergraduate/graduate classes as an Adjunct Professor at Trevecca Nazarene and Cumberland Universities.

Dirk Essary   holds a PhD in Training and Performance Improvement from Capella University and an M.B.A. from Middle Tennessee State University. He has 25 years of experience in training across corporate, government, and academic industries where his roles including training development, training management, performance improvement, and leadership. He is an Adjunct Professor for Union University. He currently is a Senior Customer Relations Manager with Vanderbilt University Medical Center.

Chapter 15
Fast Tracking Changes

Kathleen Mandato and Dirk Essary

Abstract In the healthcare world, there are frequent technology changes and updates that routinely impact key stakeholders. The learning professional is often responsible for communicating changes and providing the training that may be required. This chapter explores reasons for frequent HIT change and communication strategies that can be used to efficiently manage frequent change.

Keywords Health Information Technology · Stakeholders · Change · Upgrade · Rapid change

Learning Outcomes
1. Describe the impact of frequent HIT changes
2. List two change communication strategies
3. Demonstrate an analysis of the impact of change on different stakeholders

K. Mandato (✉)
Epic Training and Delivery and Administrative/Nursing Fellowship Program, Vanderbilt University Medical Center, Nashville, TN, USA

D. Essary
Department of Hearing and Speech Sciences, Vanderbilt University Medical Center, Nashville, TN, USA

© The Author(s), under exclusive license to Springer Nature Switzerland AG 2022
B. Kulhanek, K. Mandato (eds.), *Healthcare Technology Training*, Health Informatics, https://doi.org/10.1007/978-3-031-10322-3_15

> **The Importance of Change Communication**
> *Jennifer arrived at the hospital, ready for her next shift. She logged into the EHR and proceeded to the assessment screens to document on her first patient of the day. She sighed in frustration as she noticed the screens had been changed yet again without any prior notice! Now it was going to take extra time to figure out where to document in an already busy day!*

Key Stakeholders and Impact of Change

Technology is subject to rapid change and frequent updates. The technology used in today's home computers is exponentially more powerful than just 5 or 10 years ago. The storage capacity, processor speeds, and functional ability are all dramatically greater than before. In healthcare, workplaces continue to change and the technology used in healthcare must keep pace with technological changes, system upgrades, and user-specified practice and optimization updates.

A recent example of a required rapid change is the need to train incoming clinical labor pools and staff who have changed roles to use the EHR in preparation for an incoming surge of COVID-19 patients. In these situations, when patient care is impacted or changed, training professionals must quickly come together to determine an abbreviated method for how to train clinical staff. Adapting to this rapid change may mean streamlining existing curriculum, eliminating complexity, and removing explanatory content and interactive learning activities. In situations such as this, only the relevant content should be presented to meet the need for rapid change. To address potential knowledge gaps that could occur from abbreviated training, learning professionals may consider providing an abbreviated version of key clinical processes for job aids and in preparation for any future urgent situations.

The challenge in managing change is not always the changes themselves, but the impact of dealing with the fast pace of change and the impact on healthcare staff. As noted in Chap. 4, there are multiple models and theories that guide managing change. However, frequent and rapid change needs can occur at a pace that renders the usual change management strategies too difficult to use when fast turnaround is required.

Change Facilitation Practices

The learning professional must always remain aware of the emotional impact of change on the learner audience. Although some people embrace change and thrive in a continually changing environment, many others can become anxious or resigned. One change response framework lists a range of seven human responses to change that include aggressive resistance, active resistance, passive resistance, indifference, support, involvement, and commitment (Coetsee's Framework of Change Responses in [1]). A majority of responses to change fall into the middle five of the seven potential change responses and health care staff are more willing to accept and adopt change when certain conditions are met. Health care professionals want to know why a change is occurring and when they understand the necessity of the change they are more likely to support the change. In addition, when change was well-communicated and predictable, health care professionals are better able to prepare for the change [1].

Gaining Adoption of Rapid Change

Helping the learner accept change is key to the success of the end user. Macro changes are those that impact an entire organization and typically have the support of organizational leaders and a change management strategy. Frequent technology changes that impact smaller segments of an organization are considered micro changes. Micro changes are often primarily supported by middle and first level leaders within the organizational structure, such as managers and supervisors [2]. These mid-level leaders, as the primary stakeholders, must be familiar with ongoing changes so that they can help facilitate and support the frequent changes in their staff. Within the health care micro-culture, collective leadership, common values, and the drive towards positive change can help embed frequent change into the culture [3]. Creating change workgroups, including adding change communication in the agenda for unit councils, and developing predictable change communication paths allow each area to be able to be prepared for change and to communicate the reasons for the change to the health care professionals within their micro-culture.

Communicating Rapid Change

When creating an effective change communication pathway, the method of communication must be considered. In fact, within a single organization, there may be multiple means of communication that differ from one care area to another. Using a single change communication method typically will not meet the communication needs of all stakeholders. When the change communication pathway is being developed, stakeholders from each care area must be involved in the discussion of how communication is best delivered and received in each care area. The communication pathway must be designed so that there is a sense of importance and urgency associated with the communication. An example of a change pathway in a micro-culture is top-down communication, starting with a change communication that is sent via email to a section leader or manager. When the email is received, the manager in turn meets with the health care staff or the change team, and reviews the changes, ensuring that health care staff on all shifts are included in the communication.

It is also important to communicate the degree of importance the change represents for each area impacted by the coming change. The way a message is conveyed can drive the speed of the response to the change message. Effective communication ensures that the value and urgency of the message is conveyed along with the change facts. Changes that are of a high or critical priority, such as an emergency system downtime, may need an alternative method of communication that indicates the importance of the message. As a learning professional, part of the process of distributing communication is to understand the level of urgency and impact of a change and share the degree of importance with stakeholders, recognizing that a change of high priority in one care area may not be a high priority change in a different care area.

To ensure that all emerging and upcoming changes are included in change communication, the learning professional and team must ensure that they are connected to all of the areas within the organization where technology changes may arise, include the informatics team, the information technology (IT) team, special change groups, and senior leaders. Without an established incoming pipeline, there may be a failure to communicate significant changes that can contribute to change fatigue and further resistance to change.

Training and Rapid Changes

There are occasions when learning professionals may need to demonstrate a new process, or create education about a new process for the end users. The key to effective training is to understand how the training content will be disseminated. Again, rapid training should be distributed using a consistent method. It is also important to ensure that an organization has processes in place for rapid training, or the rapid training process may need to be examined and updated for maximum impact and distribution. Leaders are important stakeholders who must ensure that their staff are aware of, and complete the training within the established timeline. Similar to communication content, it is important to share why the change is needed and the benefits of the change. Keep in mind that the learning professional may not intuitively know the reason for a change and must investigate to make sure the correct message is communicated.

All of the best practices and time spent crafting a detailed checklist for implementing routine change may need to be set aside to pull together a miracle in a constricted timeframe. Learning professionals are often the ones who save the day through quick responses and innovation. While not ideal and certainly not recommended as normal practice, the nature of training allows for rapid analysis and deployment of resources to the targeted problem or entity. Learning professionals are used to thinking quickly on their feet and even with the best planning may have to deal with surprises such as a change in the system not previously communicated or new information that must be applied quickly to an emerging situation.

Training professionals must be as agile as possible, and ready for a rapidly changing environment. Adapting to change requires the effective use of all acquired skills. It is important to continue to build skills as a learning professional to be able to adapt successfully to change. For continued growth, the learning professional should routinely reflect on their own skill sets and abilities. When there are opportunities to develop and grow, taking the time to learn prior to a crisis can help the learning professional and the training team to be compatible with change and to successfully adapt to and manage rapid transformation.

Discussion Questions and Answers
1. What key element in training changes must a trainer be aware of and address?
   The learner's fear of change is important to keep in mind and address.
2. Who are the key stakeholders?
   The stakeholders are those who will stand to gain or lose the most because of an action. Knowing this group helps the trainer understand the importance of the change as well as who it affects.
3. What drives rapid changes?
   Most of the time it is advancing technology and the rate of improvement that drives changes in systems used in organizations.

References

1. Nilsen P, Schildmeijer K, Ericsson C, Seing I, Birken S. Implementation of change in health care in Sweden: a qualitative study of professionals' change responses. Implement Sci. 2019;14(51) https://doi.org/10.1186/s13012-019-0902-6.
2. Harden E, Ford LR, Pattie M, Lanier P. Understanding organizational change management: the role of micro and macro influences. Leadersh Organ Dev J. 2021;42(1):144–60. https://doi.org/10.1108/LODJ-01-2020-0031.
3. Sanders K, Webster J, Manley K, Cardiff S. Recognising and developing effective workplace cultures across health and social care that are also good places to work. In: International practice development in health and social care. Hoboken, NJ: Wiley-Blackwell; 2021. p. 205–19.

Kathleen Mandato is the Director of Epic Training & Delivery and the Administrative/Nursing Fellowship Program at Vanderbilt University Medical Center. She has worked in the field of training and organizational development for the last 27 years; 10 years in telecommunications, and 17 years in the healthcare industry. Kathleen has an MBA and a PhD in Education with a specialization in Training & Performance Improvement. She is a registered corporate coach and is Epic Software certified in the Cadence application. Kathleen also teaches healthcare related undergraduate/graduate classes as an Adjunct Professor at Trevecca Nazarene and Cumberland Universities.

Dirk Essary holds a PhD in Training and Performance Improvement from Capella University and an M.B.A. from Middle Tennessee State University. He has 25 years of experience in training across corporate, government, and academic industries where his roles including training development, training management, performance improvement, and leadership. He is an Adjunct Professor for Union University. He currently is a Senior Customer Relations Manager with Vanderbilt University Medical Center.

Index

Printed in the United States
by Baker & Taylor Publisher Services